Ablative Procedures in Surgical Oncology

Guest Editor

STEVEN A. CURLEY, MD

SURGICAL ONCOLOGY CLINICS OF NORTH AMERICA

www.surgonc.theclinics.com

Consulting Editor
NICHOLAS J. PETRELLI, MD

April 2011 • Volume 20 • Number 2

SAUNDERS an imprint of ELSEVIER, Inc.

W.B. SAUNDERS COMPANY
A Division of Elsevier Inc.

1600 John F. Kennedy Boulevard • Suite 1800 • Philadelphia, PA 19103-2899

http://www.theclinics.com

SURGICAL ONCOLOGY CLINICS OF NORTH AMERICA Volume 20, Number 2
April 2011 ISSN 1055-3207, ISBN-13: 978-1-4557-0511-5

Editor: Jessica Demetriou

Surgical Oncology Clinics of North America (ISSN 1055-3207) is published quarterly by Elsevier Inc., 360 Park Avenue South, New York, NY 10010-1710. Months of publication are January, April, July, and October. Business and Editorial Offices: 1600 John F. Kennedy Blvd., Ste. 1800, Philadelphia, PA 19103-2899. Customer Service Office: 3251 Riverport Lane, Maryland Heights, MO 63043. Periodicals postage paid at New York, NY and additional mailing offices. Subscription prices are $241.00 per year (US individuals), $357.00 (US institutions) $119.00 (US student/resident), $277.00 (Canadian individuals), $444.00 (Canadian institutions), $171.00 (Canadian student/resident), $346.00 (foreign individuals), $444.00 (foreign institutions), and $171.00 (foreign student/resident). Foreign air speed delivery is included in all *Clinics* subscription prices. All prices are subject to change without notice. **POSTMASTER**: Send address changes to *Surgical Oncology Clinics of North America*, Elsevier Health Science Division, Subscription Customer Service, 3251 Riverport Lane, Maryland Heights, MO 63043. **Customer Service: 1-800-654-2452 (US and Canada). 314-447-8871 (outside U.S. and Canada). Fax: 314-447-8029.** E-mail: journalscustomerservice-usa@elsevier.com (for print support); **journalsonline support-usa@elsevier.com** (for online support).

Reprints. For copies of 100 or more, of articles in this publication, please contact the Commercial Reprints Department, Elsevier Inc., 360 Park Avenue South, New York, New York 10010-1710. Tel. 212-633-3813; Fax: 212-462-1935; E-mail: reprints@elsevier.com.

Surgical Oncology Clinics of North America is covered in *MEDLINE/PubMed (Index Medicus)* and *EMBASE/ Excerpta Medica, Current Contents/Clinical Medicine,* and *ISI/BIOMED.*

Printed and bound by CPI Group (UK) Ltd, Croydon, CR0 4YY
Transferred to Digital Print 2011

Contributors

CONSULTING EDITOR

NICHOLAS J. PETRELLI, MD
Bank of America Endowed Medical Director, Helen F. Graham Cancer Center at
Christiana Care Health System, Newark, Delaware; Professor of Surgery,
Thomas Jefferson University, Philadelphia, Pennsylvania

GUEST EDITOR

STEVEN A. CURLEY, MD, FACS
Professor of Surgical Oncology, Charles B. Barker Chair in Surgery, Chief of
Gastrointestinal Tumor Surgery, The University of Texas MD Anderson Cancer Center,
Houston, Texas

AUTHORS

MUNEEB AHMED, MD
Assistant Professor of Radiology, Interventional Radiology Section/Laboratory for
Minimally Invasive Tumor Therapies, Department of Radiology, Beth Israel Deaconess
Medical Center, Harvard Medical School, Boston, Massachusetts

KAMRAN AHRAR, MD
Associate Professor, Department of Diagnostic Imaging; Medical Director, Section
of Interventional Radiology, The University of Texas MD Anderson Cancer Center,
Houston, Texas

PIYAPORN BOONSIRIKAMCHAI, MD
Research Fellow, Department of Diagnostic Radiology, The University of Texas
MD Anderson Cancer Center, Houston, Texas

CHRISTOPHER L. BRACE, PhD
Assistant Professor, Department of Radiology; Department of Biomedical Engineering,
University of Wisconsin, Madison, Wisconsin

RUSSELL E. BROWN, MD
Division of Surgical Oncology, Department of Surgery, University of Louisville, Louisville,
Kentucky

CHUSILP CHARNSANGAVEJ, MD
Professor of Radiology, Department of Diagnostic Radiology, The University of Texas
MD Anderson Cancer Center, Houston, Texas

HAESUN CHOI, MD
Professor of Radiology, Department of Diagnostic Radiology, The University of Texas
MD Anderson Cancer Center, Houston, Texas

KATHLEEN CHRISTIANS, MD
Associate Professor of Surgery, Division of Surgical Oncology, Medical College
of Wisconsin, Milwaukee, Wisconsin

STEVEN A. CURLEY, MD, FACS
Professor of Surgical Oncology, Charles B. Barker Chair in Surgery, Chief of
Gastrointestinal Tumor Surgery, The University of Texas MD Anderson Cancer Center,
Houston, Texas

T. CLARK GAMBLIN, MD, MS
Associate Professor of Surgery, Chief of Surgical Oncology, Division of Surgical
Oncology, Medical College of Wisconsin, Milwaukee, Wisconsin

EVAN S. GLAZER, MD, MPH
Research Fellow, Department of Surgical Oncology, The University of Texas
MD Anderson Cancer Center, Houston, Texas; Department of Surgery,
The University of Arizona, Tucson, Arizona

S. NAHUM GOLDBERG, MD
Professor of Radiology, Laboratory for Minimally Invasive Tumor Therapies,
Department of Radiology, Beth Israel Deaconess Medical Center, Harvard Medical
School, Boston, Massachusetts; Division of Image-Guided Therapy, Department
of Radiology, Hadassah Hebrew University Medical Center, Jerusalem, Israel

J. LOUIS HINSHAW, MD
Associate Professor, Department of Radiology, University of Wisconsin, Madison,
Wisconsin

ROSA F. HWANG, MD
Associate Professor of Surgery, Department of Surgical Oncology, The University
of Texas MD Anderson Cancer Center, Houston, Texas

JOSE A. KARAM, MD
Fellow, Department of Urology, The University of Texas MD Anderson Cancer Center,
Houston, Texas

FRED T. LEE Jr, MD
Professor, Department of Radiology, University of Wisconsin, Madison, Wisconsin

TITO LIVRAGHI, MD
Consultant, Interventional Radiology Department, Istituto Clinico Humanitas, Rozzano,
Milan, Italy

EVELYNE M. LOYER, MD
Professor of Radiology, Department of Diagnostic Radiology, The University of Texas
MD Anderson Cancer Center, Houston, Texas

MEGHAN G. LUBNER, MD
Assistant Professor, Department of Radiology, University of Wisconsin, Madison,
Wisconsin

ROBERT C.G. MARTIN II, MD, PhD
Division of Surgical Oncology, Department of Surgery, University of Louisville, Louisville,
Kentucky

SURENA F. MATIN, MD, FACS
Associate Professor, Department of Urology; Medical Director, Minimally Invasive New Technology in Oncologic Surgery (MINTOS), The University of Texas MD Anderson Cancer Center, Houston, Texas

JAVIER NAZARIO, MD
Fellow, Vascular and Interventional Radiology, The University of Texas MD Anderson Cancer Center, Houston, Texas; Interventional Radiology Department, Hospital HIMA-San Pablo, Bayamón, Puerto Rico

SAM G. PAPPAS, MD
Assistant Professor of Surgery, Division of Surgical Oncology, Medical College of Wisconsin, Milwaukee, Wisconsin

CHARLES R. SCOGGINS, MD, MBA
Division of Surgical Oncology, Department of Surgery, University of Louisville, Louisville, Kentucky

RANJNA SHARMA, MD
Instructor in Surgery, Department of Surgery, Harvard Medical School, Beth Israel Deaconess Medical Center, Boston, Massachusetts

P. DAVID SONNTAG, MD
Department of Radiology, University of Wisconsin, Madison, Wisconsin

ALDA L. TAM, MD, FRCPC, MBA
Assistant Professor, Vascular and Interventional Radiology, The University of Texas MD Anderson Cancer Center, Houston, Texas

JAMIE L. WAGNER, DO
Assistant Professor of Surgery, Department of Surgical Oncology, The University of Texas MD Anderson Cancer Center, Houston, Texas

JOHN F. WARD, MD, FACS
Assistant Professor, Department of Urology, The University of Texas MD Anderson Cancer Center, Houston, Texas

SURENA F. MATIN, MD, FACS
Associate Professor, Department of Urology, Medical Director, Minimally Invasive New Technology in Oncologic Surgery (MINTOS), The University of Texas MD Anderson Cancer Center, Houston, Texas

JAVIER NAZARIO, MD
Fellow, Vascular and Interventional Radiology, The University of Texas MD Anderson Cancer Center, Houston, Texas; Interventional Radiology Department, Hospital HIMA-San Pablo, Bayamon, Puerto Rico

SAM G. PAPPAS, MD
Associate Professor of Surgery, Department of Surgical Oncology, Medical College of Wisconsin, Milwaukee, Wisconsin

CHARLES R. ROGERS, EdD, MPH

Contents

> Through 5,000 years of practice, physicians, surgeons, clergy, or lay people have used thermal therapy to treat mass lesions now known as cancer. The methods have changed dramatically over this time span and certainly the techniques have improved the efficacy and safety. Hyperthermia used in combination with chemotherapy or ionizing radiation continues to improve outcomes. The authors briefly describe the historical role of hyperthermia in cancer care as well as modern expectations based on technological advancements. In particular, the article focuses on the role of hyperthermia for cancers that do not have other, more effective treatments.

> Thermal ablation, which induces irreversible cellular injury from focal high-temperature tissue heating that is generated from a focal energy source, has become an accepted treatment option for focal primary and secondary malignancies in a wide range of organs including the liver, lung, kidney, bone, and adrenal glands. Given the rising complexity of treatment types and paradigms in oncology, and the wider application of thermal ablation techniques and adjuvant therapy reviewed in this article, a thorough understanding of the basic principles and recent advances in thermal ablation is a necessary prerequisite for their effective clinical use.

> Ablative therapies remain a useful adjunct in the multidisciplinary treatment of patients with colorectal liver metastases not amenable to hepatic resection. This review summarizes the rationale, underlying mechanisms, techniques, complications, and outcomes of current and emerging ablative modalities.

> Neuroendocrine cancer commonly metastasizes to the liver and often presents as unresectable disease. Liver resection or debulking most of the tumor provides a survival advantage for patients. Whether used alone or in combination with resection, radiofrequency ablation provides a unique

tool to destroy metastases to the liver and spare hepatic parenchyma. Although randomized trials are lacking, retrospective series provide promising data to consider radiofrequency ablation in the management of hepatic neuroendocrine metastases.

Radiofrequency ablation (RFA), usually performed under percutaneous ultrasound guidance, is considered the gold standard among minimally invasive therapies. On the strength of some recent randomized trials, its indications include operable patients with small hepatocellular carcinoma and inoperable patients with more advanced disease also in combination with other therapies. RFA has lower complication rates and costs less than surgery.

CTs or MRIs are essential for preablative therapy planning of hepatic tumors to identify accurate size, number, and location of tumors. Tumors larger than 5 cm and located near the major branches of the portal vein and hepatic vein have a higher potential for incomplete ablation. Postablative imaging studies are needed to determine if the entire tumors are included in the treatment zone to minimize the risk of local tumor recurrences. Complications of ablative therapy can be identified on post-treatment imaging studies.

Minimally invasive ablative therapy techniques are being used in research protocols to treat benign and malignant tumors of the breast in select patient populations. These techniques offer the advantages of an outpatient setting, decreased pain, and improved cosmesis. These therapies, including radiofrequency ablation, cryotherapy, interstitial laser therapy, high-intensity focused ultrasonography, and focused microwave thermotherapy, are reviewed in this article.

While surgical excision remains the gold standard for curative treatment of small renal cell carcinomas, ablative therapy has a place as a minimally invasive, kidney function–preserving therapy in carefully selected patients who are poor candidates for surgery. Although laparoscopic cryoablation and percutaneous radiofrequency ablation (RFA) are commonly performed, percutaneous cryoablation and laparoscopic RFA are reportedly being performed with increasing frequency. The renal function and complication profiles following ablative therapy are favorable, while oncologic outcomes lag behind those of surgery, thus reinforcing the need for careful patient selection.

RELATED INTEREST

Hematology/Oncology Clinics of North America, October 2010 (Vol. 24, Issue 5)
Genetic Predisposition to Cancer
Kenneth Offit, MD, MPH, and Mark Robson, MD, *Guest Editors*
Available at: http://www.hemonc.theclinics.com/

VISIT THE CLINICS ONLINE!

Access your subscription at:
www.theclinics.com

Foreword

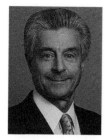

Nicholas J. Petrelli, MD
Consulting Editor

This edition of the *Surgical Oncology Clinics of North America* is devoted to "ablative procedures in surgical oncology." The guest editor is Steven A. Curley, MD. Dr Curley has been on the faculty in the Department of Surgical Oncology at The University of Texas MD Anderson Cancer Center since completing his fellowship. He is Professor of Surgical Oncology, Chief of Gastrointestinal Tumor Surgery, and Program Director of Multidisciplinary Gastrointestinal Cancer Care at MD Anderson. Dr Curley has been a pioneer in designing new treatments for patients with liver tumors, including radiofrequency ablation, improved techniques for surgical removal of liver cancers, and several types of directed tumor injection therapy. His surgical experience is evident in the article he has written for this edition of the *Surgical Oncology Clinics of North America* entitled, "The Ongoing History of Thermal Therapy for Cancer."

Dr Curley has put together an outstanding group of investigators to educate our readers about ablative procedures in oncology. Articles include ablative therapies for colorectal liver metastases, kidney tumors, and neuroendocrine hepatic metastases among others. All of these articles are a tremendous educational opportunity for residents and fellows in training, and I encourage all surgical program directors to share this particular edition of the *Surgical Oncology Clinics of North America* with their trainees. As Dr Curley states in his own article, "new technologies should permit less invasive hyperthermia therapy while noninvasive hyperthermia therapy will be a reality in the near future." I have no doubt that in view of Dr Curley's experience, in both the clinical and the research arena, that indeed his statement will become a reality in the future.

I thank Dr Curley and his associates for an outstanding edition of the *Surgical Oncology Clinics of North America*.

Nicholas J. Petrelli, MD
Helen F. Graham Cancer Center
4701 Ogletown-Stanton Road, Suite 1213
Newark, DE 19713, USA

E-mail address:
npetrelli@christianacare.org

Surg Oncol Clin N Am 20 (2011) xi
doi:10.1016/j.soc.2010.12.001
1055-3207/11/$ – see front matter © 2011 Elsevier Inc. All rights reserved.

surgonc.theclinics.com

Preface

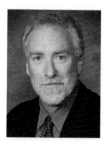

Steven A. Curley, MD
Guest Editor

In the never ending quest for new or improved ways to treat human medical disorders, mankind has used thermal therapies for thousands of years. There is evidence from ancient writings on the use of hot oils or scalding water to treat what were presumably accessible malignant tumors. Cauterization of tumors with metal probes or irons heated in fires was used during the Renaissance. In the modern era, we have continued to freeze or heat tumors in an attempt to control, and hopefully cure, malignant tumors in sites where resection is not feasible or is medically contraindicated.

In 2011, it will have been 10 years since the Food and Drug Administration approved radiofrequency ablation (RFA) as a treatment for unresectable primary or secondary liver malignancies. Since that time, there have been hundreds of articles written about RFA to treat malignant tumors of the liver, breast, thyroid, kidneys, bones, lungs, and prostate. There is now a burgeoning interest in use of microwave probes to produce thermal destruction of tumors in a more rapid fashion. All of these thermal treatments have tended to utilize local intra- and peritumoral application of freezing or heating to produce local control of malignant disease. There are limitations to the areas in the body that can be treated with thermal ablation techniques, and over the past decade a great deal has been learned about the approaches, indications, and limitations of local tumor destruction through heating. The complexity of treatment planning, particularly for larger tumors, coupled with issues regarding the requirement for concomitant imaging expertise to assure accurate placement of probes or electrodes into tumors to be treated has produced a broad spectrum of results. Incomplete thermal destruction of any part of the tumor, often erroneously reported as a local recurrence, represents a failure to produce temperature extremes through all areas of the tumor sufficient to produce apoptosis or necrosis of all malignant cells.

In this issue of the *Surgical Oncology Clinics of North America* there are some excellent reviews on the state of knowledge of the use of thermal therapies to treat malignant disease. Drs Ahmed and Goldberg have provided a thorough and rigorous review of the state of basic science research in thermal ablation techniques. This includes issues in imaging, thermal conductivity in tissues, and distribution of heat adequate to produce complete control of a malignant lesion. The next three articles review the use of ablative therapies to treat colorectal cancer liver metastases,

Surg Oncol Clin N Am 20 (2011) xiii–xiv
doi:10.1016/j.soc.2010.12.002
1055-3207/11/$ – see front matter © 2011 Elsevier Inc. All rights reserved.

surgonc.theclinics.com

neuroendocrine cancer liver metastases, and primary hepatocellular carcinoma, respectively. This includes considerations with use of both RFA and microwave ablation of malignant liver tumors. Finishing out the information regarding thermal therapies for hepatic tumors is an article on treatment planning with state-of-the-art hepatic imaging, as well as a treatise on the radiographic findings in tumors treated with thermal ablation techniques.

The second set of articles in this issue deals with ablative therapies for malignant tumors of the breast, kidneys, bones, and lungs, respectively. While the experience with thermal therapy for tumors in these body sites is not as extensive as for hepatic malignancies, there is definitely a role in properly selected patients for the use of these local tumor destruction techniques. Unfortunately, as is true in other areas of surgical practice, there is a paucity or absence of prospective randomized studies to evaluate rigorously the role of thermal therapies compared to standard surgical resections or other alternative treatments.

The final article by Dr Ward provides a thorough review of the use of high-intensity focused ultrasound for ablation of malignant tissues. This technique is gaining increased exposure and experience worldwide and promises to add another tool in the armamentarium for surgical oncologists interested in alternative or additive treatments to their surgical techniques.

Surgeons have long been at the forefront of investigations to improve the safety and effectiveness of cancer control. While thermal tumor ablation techniques have been used for centuries, the techniques and equipment continue to evolve and improve. Local tumor ablation techniques, like surgical resection, are designed to provide local control of malignant disease in a variety of organ sites. Those of us who use these local tumor ablation techniques have seen an increase in the number of patients in whom we can successfully control their malignant disease and produce long-term quality survival. We are now seeing not only 5-year survivors, but individuals who have survived greater than 10 years after thermal ablation of malignant disease. Unfortunately, this continues to be too few patients because of the systemic nature of malignant disease. Thus, further research and evaluation of multidisciplinary approaches to treat patients with malignant tumors, which include the application of local thermal therapies, will be critical in the next few years.

Steven A. Curley, MD
Department of Surgical Oncology
The University of Texas MD Anderson Cancer Center
Unit 444, Office FC12.3058
1400 Holcombe Boulevard
Houston, TX 77030, USA

E-mail address:
scurley@mdanderson.org

The Ongoing History of Thermal Therapy for Cancer

Evan S. Glazer, MD, MPH[a,b], Steven A. Curley, MD[a,*]

KEYWORDS

- Thermal therapy • Ablative techniques • Hyperthermia
- Electrotherapy

Hyperthermia has been used with an "intent to cure" tumors for at least 4000 years, and as a tool for the destruction of tumor masses well before that.[1] Tumors refer to any growth or mass that has developed unexpectedly. Well before there was any understanding of the molecular basis for cancer, let alone the ability to diagnose cancer, there was an understanding that cutting or burning of these lesions was an appropriate therapy for some affected individuals. In fact, Hippocrates[1,2] describes that if a tumor "cannot be cut, it should burned. If it cannot be burned, then it is incurable." However shocking, for many cancers this is still the case.

While chemotherapy may "cure" a few fortunate patients with various types of cancer, malignant diseases such as metastatic hepatocellular carcinoma (HCC) are usually incurable, with no meaningful 5-year survival probability in the majority of patients. In other patients who have locally advanced unresectable hepatic lesions, radiofrequency (RF) thermal ablation is a useful and potentially curative therapy for HCC. Notwithstanding the few patients who have some benefit from transhepatic arterial embolization, there is no curative systemic or regional cytotoxic chemotherapy for HCC. The most recently approved targeted therapy for HCC, sorafenib, increases median survival of patients with unresectable HCC by 3 months.[3] Patients with unresectable metastatic lesions (such as colorectal cancer) to the liver that are amenable to RF ablation have a median overall survival of 25 to 30 months, in general.[4]

The authors have nothing to disclose.

E.S.G. is an NIH T32 research fellow (T32 CA09599). This research is supported in part by the National Institutes of Health through the University of Texas MD Anderson's Cancer Center Support Grant CA016672.

Conflicts of interest. The authors declare that there are no conflicts of interest.

[a] Department of Surgical Oncology, The University of Texas MD Anderson Cancer Center, Unit 444, Office FC12.3058, 1400 Holcombe Boulevard, Houston, TX 77030, USA

[b] Department of Surgery, The University of Arizona, 1501 North Campbell Avenue, PO Box 245058, Tucson, AZ 85724-5058, USA

* Corresponding author.

E-mail address: scurley@mdanderson.org

There are multiple forms of hyperthermic therapy. The aforementioned RF ablation technique is a local therapy involving intratumoral placement of a needle electrode that can produce tissue temperatures as high as 100°C following activation of an electrical current. Alternating electrical current dissipation and ionic stimulation within tissue surrounding the electrode causes hyperthermia. Regional hyperthermia has been used in combination with regional chemotherapy during resection of extremity soft tissue sarcomas or as treatment for in-transit limb metastases from melanoma.[5] In these cases, the elevated tissue temperature is maintained for extended periods of time. This procedure takes the form of an isolated limb perfusion of chemotherapy warmed to 42°C to 45°C for 60 minutes or longer.[5] Likewise, hyperthermic intraperitoneal chemotherapy is another regional hyperthermic treatment often performed simultaneously with resection of peritoneal malignant disease.[6] Finally, whole body hyperthermic therapy has been used by inducing fevers with toxins[7] or externally warming entire patients up to 42°C for extended periods of time.[8,9]

It is often quoted that Hippocrates "managed" superficial tumors with cautery or direct ablative therapy, but it is not clear if he was actually describing the treatment of cancer.[1] It is interesting that the side effects he mentions include weakness, neurologic changes, hemorrhage, and death, which are all adverse events that are similar to what is seen today with whole body hyperthermic treatment.[1,9,10] Around the Middle Ages and later, instruments were designed and shaped for direct application of heat to kill tumors or cauterize bleeding, albeit without the benefit of adequate regional or general anesthesia (**Fig. 1**).

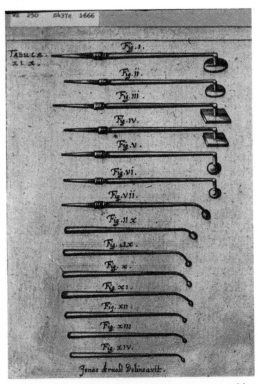

Fig. 1. Fourteen different instruments used for cautery as engraved by Jonas Arnold Deliveavit (ca 1666). This image was acquired from The National Library of Medicine's *Images from the History of Medicine* collection in the public domain.

Finally, the goal of hyperthermic therapy is to capitalize on the difference in thermo-tolerance between normal and cancer cells.[11] Mammalian cells die when exposed to temperatures above 55°C for more than a few minutes; however, these normal cells tolerate temperature ranges from 41°C to 43°C for hours. Of importance, each half of a degree increase in cellular temperature is associated with increased cell death. Cancer cells in general do not tolerate these temperatures nearly as well or as long. Finding the appropriate balance of temperature and duration is finding the balance between the desired cancer cell death and undesirable normal cell toxicity.

EARLY ELECTROSURGERY

Electrosurgical procedures in the first half of the twentieth century included destruction of cancerous tissues, enlarged lymph nodes, and cauterization of nodules left after enucleation of other masses.[12,13] Of note, these included intra-abdominal procedures of the uterus and ovaries[12] as well as intrathoracic procedures for cancers and infections.[13] In 1900, the first modern example of curative electrosurgery for cancer was documented when an artist who had a cutaneous carcinoma accidently touched an electrical wire. The current "treated" his cutaneous carcinoma via hyperthermia, and the concept of electrofulguration was born.[14] Soon thereafter, William T. Bovie and Harvey Cushing developed and clinically implemented an electrosurgical device for decreasing intraoperative blood loss.[14] Hyperthermic electrothermal ablation can directly trace its history to this moment.

DEVELOPMENT OF MODERN TECHNIQUES

Modern ablative techniques require direct contact between a probe, the target tumor, and surrounding normal tissue. Depending on the modality and intensity of treatment, there is an immediate zone of intratumoral necrosis, a zone of apoptosis, and a zone of hyperemia without frank cell death.[15] Ideally, there will be a margin of normal tissue death to ensure the death of all cancer cells.[4] Among many extremely well-conducted studies and reviews during the 1970s investigating the effects of hyperthermia on normal and cancer cells, a review article by Field and Bleehen described the current understanding of hyperthermia in the treatment of cancer that remains accurate to this day.[16]

Effective local or regional hyperthermic cancer therapy can be induced by either longer heating durations at temperatures of 41°C to 45°C or by short-duration treatment of cancer cells with higher temperatures (or both).[17] Likewise, many, but not all, cancer cells respond differently from their normal cell origins to hyperthermic therapy.[16] The difference between these 2 responses permits a general method to treat cancers with hyperthermia. This is not to suggest that all cancers can be treated in the same manner, but this approach has worked well in RF ablation of primary and secondary liver malignancies.[18] The approach is to maximize the coagulative necrosis of the malignancy in situ while accepting limited necrosis or apoptosis of surrounding normal parenchyma. In this way, excess normal tissue is not needlessly injured while "oncologically" safe margins are maintained. Furthermore, all cancer cells are presumed to be within the area of coagulative necrosis and are immediately killed during the procedure. The balance of treatment effectiveness, patient safety, and normal hepatocyte tolerance resulted in a nearly uniform practice of treating properly selected hepatic tumors for approximately 10 minutes with tissue temperatures of at least 60°C to 65°C.[4]

More recent examples of direct electrosurgery are seen in the practice of endobronchial procedures and cervical lesions.[19–21] Whereas loop electrosurgical procedures are standard therapy for premalignant cervical lesions, at present endobronchial ablative therapy is not standard for cancers of the upper airways. However, it provides interesting and effective use of hyperthermic cautery based on the principles previously described. Of note, complete excision of premalignant or early malignant cervical lesions confers extremely high rates of cure for a disease, much like HCC, that otherwise carries a very poor prognosis when it is found to be advanced.[22–24]

MODERN ABLATIVE TECHNIQUES

RF ablation of unresectable metastatic hepatic colorectal malignancies is the prototypical local tumor ablative procedure.[25] Likewise, RF ablation for primary hepatocellular carcinoma, neuroendocrine hepatic metastases, and other unresectable hepatic lesions is very common.[26] Often, RF ablation is performed synchronously with hepatic resection, the gold standard for surgical management of primary and secondary liver malignancies.[25,27] Finally, management of esophageal dysplastic lesions can often be safely managed with RF ablation.[28]

Microwave ablation, which has been very useful in Europe and Asia for many years, is slowly becoming more popular in the United States.[29] Whereas monopolar RF ablation works by inducing an alternating electrical current from the probe to the tumor with excess energy dissipated through the patient to large grounding pads, microwave ablation works by exploiting rapid oscillation of water molecules based on the dipole moment of water around a microwave-emitting probe(s). The current in RF ablation passes via the path of least resistance, potentially resulting in asymmetric ablation patterns. Microwave ablation, however, will destroy anything within the confines of the field for a given treatment duration and power, including a potentially higher risk to damage normal tissues such as bile ducts and vascular structures.[29,30]

Cryoablation is the technique of using extremely cold probes to bring the temperatures of surrounding tumors to below the cytotoxic freezing threshold (< approximately −20°C to as cold as −130°C) for up to 10 minutes with subsequent active heating for typically 2 to 3 cycles.[31,32] Although systems vary, most use the conversion of high-pressure gas to cold low-pressure liquid to reach these extremely low temperatures. The urologic oncology community uses cryoablation more so than RF ablation to treat prostate cancer,[33,34] while there is evidence that in hepatic lesions, RF ablation is more effective than cryoablation.[35–37]

FUTURE DIRECTIONS

While invasive RF ablation remains the standard of care in the United States, many surgeons expect that intratumoral probe microwave ablation will become a second standard therapy for unresectable cancers. Unfortunately, microwave ablation rapidly produces excessive heat that potentially destroys everything within its field, and as such is not appropriate for use near vital, critical structures such as the biliary confluence or the ureter. However, as research investigates better ways to protect these important structures, the role of microwave ablation will certainly increase.

Two "futuristic" treatments are noninvasive nanoparticle-mediated intracellular hyperthermic cytotoxicity and irreversible electroporation (IRE). Gold and gold-based nanoparticles are in preclinical and early clinical development as a means to induce targeted hyperthermia.[38–40] Through the use of near-infrared lasers or nonionizing RF fields, multiple groups have demonstrated high specificity for killing targeted cancer cells in vitro and in vivo.[39,41–43] While there are some ongoing clinical trials investigating the use of nanoparticle-induced hyperthermia as a targeted cancer treatment, this therapy is still a few years away from being available for clinical trials.

IRE is the technique of placing electrodes on either side of the lesion in situ and inducing an electric field between them.[36,44] Appropriately constructed electric fields will permanently create cell membrane defects (ie, pores) that result in cell death without hyperthermic injury. Similar to microwave ablation, any cell within the electroporation volume will die, but acellular structures (extracellular components of bile ducts) should remain intact as there is not a potential across them. IRE devices are available in the United States, but studies are ongoing.

Finally, high-intensity focused ultrasound is 10 to 1000 times more intense than diagnostic ultrasound.[45,46] Targeted tissues (ie, the ultrasound probe is focused on a tumor) absorb high-intensity acoustic energy that is converted to heat. Coagulative necrosis is typically achieved within a few seconds.[36] Early-phase trials are ongoing for HCC, prostate, and other cancers.

SUMMARY

The history of ablative therapies for cancers has been one of increasing the efficiency and specificity of treatment, not necessarily drastically changing the goals of the treatment per se. From the time of antiquity, when a heated probe cauterized a skin lesion, to today where an intratumoral needle electrode passes electricity to a liver lesion, the challenge has always remained to kill the cancer without harming the patient. New technologies should permit less invasive hyperthermic therapy while noninvasive hyperthermic therapy will be a reality in the near future. Whereas today we treat cancers with invasive local or regional hyperthermia techniques, it is not unreasonable to suggest that in the future we will manage cancers with targeted noninvasive hyperthermia.

ACKNOWLEDGMENTS

The authors would like to thank Kristine K. Ash and Jose Javier Garza for administrative assistance.

REFERENCES

1. Hornback NB. Historical aspects of hyperthermia in cancer therapy. Radiol Clin North Am 1989;27(3):481–8.
2. Hippocrates. On the articulations. The genuine works of Hippocrates. Clin Orthop Relat Res 2002;400:19–25.
3. Llovet JM, Ricci S, Mazzaferro V, et al. Sorafenib in advanced hepatocellular carcinoma. N Engl J Med 2008;359(4):378–90.
4. Curley SA, Izzo F. Radiofrequency ablation of primary and metastatic hepatic malignancies. Int J Clin Oncol 2002;7(2):72–81.
5. Issels RD, Lindner LH, Verweij J, et al. Neo-adjuvant chemotherapy alone or with regional hyperthermia for localised high-risk soft-tissue sarcoma: a randomised phase 3 multicentre study. Lancet Oncol 2010;11(6):561–70.
6. Verwaal VJ, van Ruth S, de Bree E, et al. Randomized trial of cytoreduction and hyperthermic intraperitoneal chemotherapy versus systemic chemotherapy and palliative surgery in patients with peritoneal carcinomatosis of colorectal cancer. J Clin Oncol 2003;21(20):3737–43.
7. Meyer JL. Hyperthermia as an anticancer modality—a historical perspective. Front Radiat Ther Oncol 1984;18:1–22.

8. Robins HI, Cohen JD, Schmitt CL, et al. Phase I clinical trial of carboplatin and 41.8 degrees C whole-body hyperthermia in cancer patients. J Clin Oncol 1993;11(9):1787–94.
9. Bull JM, Scott GL, Strebel FR, et al. Fever-range whole-body thermal therapy combined with cisplatin, gemcitabine, and daily interferon-alpha: a description of a phase I-II protocol. Int J Hyperthermia 2008;24(8):649–62.
10. Atmaca A, Al-Batran SE, Neumann A, et al. Whole-body hyperthermia (WBH) in combination with carboplatin in patients with recurrent ovarian cancer—a phase II study. Gynecol Oncol 2009;112(2):384–8.
11. Wust P, Nadobny J, Szimtenings M, et al. Implications of clinical RF hyperthermia on protection limits in the RF range. Health Phys 2007;92(6):565–73.
12. Kelly HA. Electrosurgery in gynaecology. Ann Surg 1931;93(1):323–5.
13. Lilienthal H. Electrosurgery: a clinical report on 118 operations. Ann Surg 1933;97(6):801–7.
14. O'Connor JL, Bloom DA, William T. Bovie and electrosurgery. Surgery 1996;119(4):390–6.
15. Curley SA. Radiofrequency ablation of malignant liver tumors. Oncologist 2001;6(1):14–23.
16. Field SB, Bleehen NM. Hyperthermia in the treatment of cancer. Cancer Treat Rev 1979;6(2):63–94.
17. Westra A, Dewey WC. Variation in sensitivity to heat shock during the cell-cycle of Chinese hamster cells in vitro. Int J Radiat Biol Relat Stud Phys Chem Med 1971;19(5):467–77.
18. Curley SA. Radiofrequency ablation of malignant liver tumors. Ann Surg Oncol 2003;10(4):338–47.
19. Emam M, Elnashar A, Shalan H, et al. Evaluation of a single-step diagnosis and treatment of premalignant cervical lesion by LEEP. Int J Gynaecol Obstet 2009;107(3):224–7.
20. Kietpeerakool C, Suprasert P, Khunamornpong S, et al. "Top hat" versus conventional loop electrosurgical excision procedure in women with a type 3 transformation zone. Int J Gynaecol Obstet 2009;109(1):59–62.
21. Duhamel DR, Harrell JH 2nd. Laser bronchoscopy. Chest Surg Clin N Am 2001;11(4):769–89.
22. Sankaranarayanan R, Keshkar V, Kothari A, et al. Effectiveness and safety of loop electrosurgical excision procedure for cervical neoplasia in rural India. Int J Gynaecol Obstet 2009;104(2):95–9.
23. Rema P, Suchetha S, Thara S, et al. Effectiveness and safety of loop electrosurgical excision procedure in a low-resource setting. Int J Gynaecol Obstet 2008;103(2):105–10.
24. Chirenje ZM, Rusakaniko S, Akino V, et al. A randomised clinical trial of loop electrosurgical excision procedure (LEEP) versus cryotherapy in the treatment of cervical intraepithelial neoplasia. J Obstet Gynaecol 2001;21(6):617–21.
25. Pawlik TM, Izzo F, Cohen DS, et al. Combined resection and radiofrequency ablation for advanced hepatic malignancies: results in 172 patients. Ann Surg Oncol 2003;10(9):1059–69.
26. Mayo SC, Pawlik TM. Thermal ablative therapies for secondary hepatic malignancies. Cancer J 2010;16(2):111–7.
27. Abdalla EK, Vauthey JN, Ellis LM, et al. Recurrence and outcomes following hepatic resection, radiofrequency ablation, and combined resection/ablation for colorectal liver metastases. Ann Surg 2004;239(6):818–27.

28. Shaheen NJ, Frantz DJ. When to consider endoscopic ablation therapy for Barrett's esophagus. Curr Opin Gastroenterol 2010;26(4):361–6.
29. Martin RC, Scoggins CR, McMasters KM. Safety and efficacy of microwave ablation of hepatic tumors: a prospective review of a 5-year experience. Ann Surg Oncol 2009;17(1):171–8.
30. Bhardwaj N, Strickland AD, Ahmad F, et al. Microwave ablation for unresectable hepatic tumours: clinical results using a novel microwave probe and generator. Eur J Surg Oncol 2009;36(3):264–8.
31. DeCastro GJ, Gupta M, Badani K, et al. Synchronous cryoablation of multiple renal lesions: short-term follow-up of patient outcomes. Urology 2009;75(2):303–6.
32. Saksena M, Gervais D. Percutaneous renal tumor ablation. Abdom Imaging 2009;34(5):582–7.
33. Gontero P, Joniau S, Zitella A, et al. Ablative therapies in the treatment of small renal tumors: how far from standard of care? Urol Oncol 2009;28(3):251–9.
34. Mouraviev V, Joniau S, Van Poppel H, et al. Current status of minimally invasive ablative techniques in the treatment of small renal tumours. Eur Urol 2007;51(2):328–36.
35. Jansen MC, van Hillegersberg R, Schoots IG, et al. Cryoablation induces greater inflammatory and coagulative responses than radiofrequency ablation or laser induced thermotherapy in a rat liver model. Surgery 2010;147(5):686–95.
36. Padma S, Martinie JB, Iannitti DA. Liver tumor ablation: percutaneous and open approaches. J Surg Oncol 2009;100(8):619–34.
37. Khan NA, Baerlocher MO, Owen RJ, et al. Ablative technologies in the management of patients with primary and secondary liver cancer: an overview. Can Assoc Radiol J 2010;61(4):217–22.
38. Cobley CM, Au L, Chen J, et al. Targeting gold nanocages to cancer cells for photothermal destruction and drug delivery. Expert Opin Drug Deliv 2010;7(5):577–87.
39. Goodrich GP, Bao L, Gill-Sharp K, et al. Photothermal therapy in a murine colon cancer model using near-infrared absorbing gold nanorods. J Biomed Opt 2010;15(1):018001.
40. Cherukuri P, Glazer ES, Curley SA. Targeted hyperthermia using metal nanoparticles. Adv Drug Deliv Rev 2010;62(3):339–45.
41. Curley SA, Cherukuri P, Briggs K, et al. Noninvasive radiofrequency field-induced hyperthermic cytotoxicity in human cancer cells using cetuximab-targeted gold nanoparticles. J Exp Ther Oncol 2008;7(4):313–26.
42. Glazer ES, Curley SA. Radiofrequency field-induced thermal cytotoxicity in cancer cells treated with fluorescent nanoparticles. Cancer 2010;116(13):3285–93.
43. El-Sayed IH. Nanotechnology in head and neck cancer: the race is on. Curr Oncol Rep 2010;12(2):121–8.
44. Al-Sakere B, Andre F, Bernat C, et al. Tumor ablation with irreversible electroporation. PLoS One 2007;2(11):e1135.
45. Fischer K, Gedroyc W, Jolesz FA. Focused ultrasound as a local therapy for liver cancer. Cancer J 2010;16(2):118–24.
46. Margreiter M, Marberger M. Focal therapy and imaging in prostate and kidney cancer: high-intensity focused ultrasound ablation of small renal tumors. J Endourol 2010;24(5):745–8.

Basic Science Research in Thermal Ablation

Muneeb Ahmed, MD[a],*, S. Nahum Goldberg, MD[a,b]

KEYWORDS

• Thermal ablation • Bioheat equation
• Minimally invasive surgery • Radiofrequency

Thermal ablation has become an accepted treatment option for focal primary and secondary malignancies in a wide range of organs including the liver, lung, kidney, bone, and adrenal glands.[1-6] The largest clinical experience has been for hepatic malignancies, where long-term outcomes similar to surgical resection have been reported in some matched patient populations.[7] Benefits of minimally invasive, image-guided ablative techniques include reduced cost and morbidity compared with standard surgical resection, and the ability to treat patients who are not surgical candidates. However, limitations in thermal ablative efficacy exist, including persistent growth of residual tumor at the ablation margin, the inability to effectively treat larger tumors, and variability in complete treatment based on tumor location. Extensive investigation into potential strategies to improve ablation outcomes continues, and focuses on technological development of ablative systems, improving ablative predictability, and combining thermal ablation with additional therapies such as chemotherapy and radiation. Given the rising complexity of treatment types and paradigms in oncology, and the wider application of thermal ablation techniques, a thorough understanding of the basic principles and recent advances in thermal ablation is a necessary prerequisite for their effective clinical use.

GOALS OF MINIMALLY INVASIVE THERMAL TUMOR ABLATION

The overall goal of minimally invasive thermal tumor ablation for focal malignancies encompasses several specific objectives, regardless of the specific thermal ablative device that is used. The primary purpose of treatment is to completely eradicate all viable malignant cells within the target tumor. Based on tumor recurrence patterns in long-term studies in patients who have undergone surgical resection, and more

---

[a] Laboratory for Minimally Invasive Tumor Therapies, Department of Radiology, Beth Israel Deaconess Medical Center, Harvard Medical School, 1 Deaconess Road, WCC 308-B, Boston, MA 02215, USA
[b] Division of Image-Guided Therapy, Department of Radiology, Hadassah Hebrew University Medical Center, Jerusalem, Israel
* Corresponding author.
E-mail address: mahmed@bidmc.harvard.edu

Surg Oncol Clin N Am 20 (2011) 237–258
doi:10.1016/j.soc.2010.11.011
1055-3207/11/$ – see front matter © 2011 Elsevier Inc. All rights reserved.

recently, ablation, along with studies that have performed pathologic analysis of resection margins, there is often viable persistent microscopic tumor foci in a rim of apparently normal surrounding parenchymal tissue beyond the visible tumor margin. Therefore, tumor ablation therapies also attempt to include a 5- to 10-mm "ablative" margin of normal surrounding tissue in the target zone, though the required thickness of this margin is variable based on tumor and organ type.[8,9] While complete treatment of the target tumor is of primary importance, specificity and accuracy is also highly preferred, with a secondary goal of incurring as little injury as possible to surrounding nontarget normal tissue. This ability to minimize damage to normal organ parenchyma is one of the significant advantages of minimally invasive percutaneous thermal ablation, and can be critical in patients who have focal tumors in the setting of limited functional organ reserve. Examples of clinical situations where this is relevant include focal hepatic tumors in patients with underlying cirrhosis and limited hepatic reserve, patients with Von Hippel Lindau syndrome who have limited renal function and require treatment of multiple renal tumors, and patients with primary lung tumors with extensive underlying emphysema and limited lung function.[10–12] Many of these patients are not surgical candidates because of limited native organ functional reserve placing them at a higher risk for postoperative complications or organ failure. An additional consideration is that appropriate and complete tumor destruction occurs only when the entire target tumor is exposed to appropriate temperatures, and is therefore determined by the pattern of tissue heating in the target tumor. For larger tumors (usually defined to be larger than 3–5 cm in diameter), a single ablation treatment may not be sufficient to entirely encompass the target volume.[3] In these cases, multiple overlapping ablations or simultaneous use of multiple applicators may be required to successfully treat the entire tumor and achieve an ablative margin, although accurate targeting and probe placement can often be technically challenging (**Fig. 1**).[13] Finally, growth patterns of the tumor itself can influence overall treatment outcomes, with slow-growing tumors more amenable to multiple treatment sessions over longer periods of time. These principles are applicable to a wide range of ablative technologies, including both thermal and nonthermal strategies.

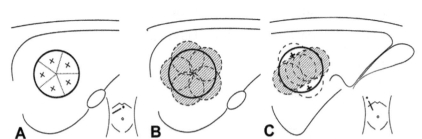

Fig. 1. Performance of multiple overlapping ablations to completely treat a large tumor, using a regular 5-sided prism model. (*A*) Maximum transverse view of the tumor: Five target sites are determined to guide electrode insertions. (*B*) Same section as *A*. Five ablations are performed in the middle part of the tumor. (*C*) The section perpendicular to *A*. Two additional ablations are performed at the 2 poles of the tumor. The tumor can be effectively ablated with 7 ablation spheres. Crosses indicate the target site of the ablation—that is, the ablation sphere center. (*From* Chen MH, Yang W, Yan K, et al. Large liver tumors: protocol for radiofrequency ablation and its clinical application in 110 patients—mathematic model, overlapping mode, and electrode placement process. Radiology 2004;232:263; with permission.)

PRINCIPLES OF TISSUE HEATING IN THERMAL ABLATION

Thermal ablation induces irreversible cellular injury from focal high-temperature tissue heating that is generated from a focal energy source. Multiple energy sources have been used to provide the heat necessary to induce coagulation necrosis. Focal high temperature (generally accepted as >50°C) ablation therapies use radiofrequency (RF), microwave, laser, or ultrasound energies to generate isolated increases in tissue temperature. Historically, the majority of clinical and experimental studies have been performed using RF-based ablative devices. As such, this review of basic principles of focal high temperature ablative therapies will primarily use RF systems as a representative model in describing the basic principles of focal thermal ablation, with discussions of other energy-based technologies where relevant.

Tissue heating occurs though 2 specific mechanisms. First, an applicator placed within the center of the target tumor delivers energy that interacts with tissue to generate focal heat immediately around it. This approach is similar for all thermal ablation strategies, regardless of the type of energy source used, though specific mechanisms of heat induction are energy specific.[14] For example, as RF current travels from the electrode applicator to the remote grounding pad, local tissue resistance to current flow results in ionic agitation and heat generation. In microwave-based systems, the needle antenna applies electromagnetic energy to the tissue, and as molecules with an intrinsic dipole moment (such as water) are forced to continuously align to the externally applied magnetic field, the kinetic energy that is generated results in local tissue heating. Laser ablation uses emission of laser energy from optic fibers to generate tissue heat immediately around the fiber tip. Ultrasound-based systems induce tissue heating by applying a focused beam of ultrasound energy with a high peak intensity, either directly around a percutaneously placed applicator (like for other ablative systems), or transcutaneously by directing several ultrasound beams of lower intensity from different directions so that they converge at the target tumor, where the ultrasound energy is absorbed by the tissue and converted to heat. The second mechanism of tissue heating in thermal ablation uses thermal tissue conduction.[15] Heat generated around the electrode diffuses through the tumor and results in additional high-temperature heating that is separate from the direct energy-tissue interactions that occur around the electrode. The contribution of thermal conduction to overall tissue ablation is determined by several factors. Tissue heating patterns vary based on the specific energy source used—for example, microwave-based systems induce tissue heating at a much faster rate than RF-based systems, and so thermal conduction contributes less to overall tissue heating.[15] In addition, tumor and tissue characteristics also affect thermal conduction. As an example, primary hepatic tumors (hepatocellular carcinoma) transmit heat better than the surrounding cirrhotic hepatic parenchyma.[3,16]

Regardless of the energy source used, the end point of thermal ablation is adequate tissue heating so as to induce coagulative necrosis throughout the defined target area. Relatively mild increases in tissue temperature above baseline (40°C) can be tolerated by normal cellular homeostatic mechanisms. Low-temperature hyperthermia (42°C–45°C) results in reversible cellular injury, though this can increase cellular susceptibility to additional adjuvant therapies such as chemotherapy and radiation.[17,18] Irreversible cellular injury occurs when cells are heated to 46°C for 60 minutes, and occurs more rapidly as the temperature rises, so that most cell types die in a few minutes when heated at 50°C.[19] Immediate cellular damage centers on protein coagulation of cytosolic and mitochondrial enzymes and nucleic acid-histone protein complexes, which triggers cellular death over the course of several days.[20] "Heat fixation" or "coagulation necrosis" is used to describe this thermal damage, even though ultimate manifestations of cell death may not fulfill strict histopathologic criteria of coagulative necrosis.[21] This has implications with regard to clinical practice, as percutaneous biopsy and standard histopathologic interpretation may not be a reliable measure of adequate ablation.[21] Therefore, optimal temperatures for ablation range likely exceed 50°C. At the other end of the temperature spectrum, tissue vaporization occurs at temperatures higher than 110°C, which in turn limits further current deposition in RF-based systems (as compared with, for example, microwave systems that do not have this limitation).

The exact temperature at which cell death occurs is multifactorial and tissue specific. Based on prior studies demonstrating that tissue coagulation can be induced by focal tissue heating to 50°C for 4 to 6 minutes,[22] this has become the standard surrogate end point for thermal ablation therapies in both experimental studies and current clinical paradigms. However, studies have shown that depending on heating time, the rate of heat increase, and the tissue being heated, maximum temperatures at the edge of ablation are variable. For example, maximum temperatures at the edge of ablation zone, known as the "critical temperature," have been shown to range from 30°C to 77°C for normal tissues and from 41°C to 64°C for tumor models (a 23°C difference).[23,24] Likewise, the total amount of heat administered for a given time, known as the thermal dose, varies significantly between different tissues.[23,24] Thus, the threshold target temperature of 50°C should be used only as a general guideline.

APPLYING THE PRINCIPLES OF THE BIOHEAT EQUATION TO ACHIEVE MEANINGFUL VOLUMES OF TUMOR ABLATION

Early studies using RF-based systems demonstrated that percutaneous thermal ablation with a single-electrode system was inadequate for tumors larger than 1.8 cm.[25] Subsequent investigation (such as the techniques described later) has increased the size of consistently achievable ablation to at least 3 to 5 cm in diameter.[3] However, with the continued expansion of the use of thermal ablation techniques into new tumor types, and the growing need for effective alternative treatment options in patients with larger tumors and who are ineligible for surgery, the need to reliably ablate larger tumors persists.

Complete and adequate destruction by thermal ablation requires that the entire tumor (and usually an ablative margin) be subjected to cytotoxic temperatures. Success of thermal ablation is contingent on adequate heat delivery. The ability to heat large volumes of tissue in different environments is dependent on several factors encompassing both energy delivery and local physiologic tissue characteristics. The relationship between this set of parameters, as described by the Bioheat equation,[26] can be simplified to describe the basic relationship guiding thermal ablation–induced coagulation necrosis as: "coagulation necrosis = (energy deposited × local tissue interactions) − heat loss."[27] Based on this relationship, several strategies to increase the ability to ablate larger tumors have been concurrently pursued. These encompass (1) technological developments, including modification of energy input algorithms and electrode design to deposit more energy into the tissue, (2) improved understanding and subsequent modification of the biophysiologic environment to increase tissue heating, and (3) incorporation of adjuvant therapies to increase uniformity of tumor cellular injury in the ablation zone, along with increasing cellular destruction in the nonlethal hyperthermic zone around the ablation.

TECHNOLOGIC ADVANCEMENTS

Most investigation to improve thermal ablation outcomes has focused on device development, much of which has been, as noted, for RF-based ablation systems. Technologic efforts to increase ablation size have focused on modifying energy deposition algorithms and electrode designs to increase both the amount of tissue exposed to the active electrode and the overall amount of energy that can be safely deposited into the target tissue.

Refinement of Energy Application Algorithms

The algorithm by which energy is applied during thermal ablation is dependent on the energy source, device, and type of electrode that is being used. While initial power algorithms for RF-based systems were based on a continuous and constant high-energy input, tissue overheating and vaporization ultimately interferes with continued energy input because of high impedance to current flow from gas formation. Therefore, several strategies to maximize energy deposition have been developed and, in some cases, incorporated into commercially available devices.

Applying high levels of energy in a pulsed manner, separated by periods of lower energy, is one such strategy that has been used with RF-based systems to increase the mean intensity of energy deposition.[28] If a proper balance between high and low energy deposition is achieved, preferential tissue cooling occurs adjacent to the electrode during periods of minimal energy deposition without significantly decreasing heating deeper in the tissue. Thus, even greater energy can be applied during periods of high energy deposition, thereby enabling deeper heat penetration and greater tissue coagulation.[29] Synergy between a combination of internal cooling of the electrode and pulsing has resulted in even greater coagulation necrosis and tumor destruction than either method alone.[29] Pulsed-energy techniques have also been successfully used for microwave and laser-based systems.

Another strategy is to slowly increase (or "ramp-up") the RF energy application in a continuous manner, until the impedance to RF current flow increases prohibitively.[30] This approach is often paired with multitined expandable electrodes, which have a greater contact surface area with tissue, and in which the goal is to achieve smaller ablation zones around multiple small electrode tines. This algorithm is also often combined with a staged expansion of the electrode system such that each small ablation occurs in a slightly different location within the tumor (with the overall goal being ablating the entire target region).

"Electrode switching" is an additional technique that is incorporated into pulsing algorithms to further increase RF tissue heating.[31] In this, multiple independently placed RF electrodes are connected to a single RF generator, and RF current is applied to a single electrode until an impedance spike is detected, at which point current application is applied to the next electrode, and so forth. Several studies have demonstrated significant increases in ablation zone size and a reduction in application time using this technique.[31,32] For example, Brace and colleagues[31] also show larger and more circular ablation zones with the switching application, with more rapid heating being 74% faster than the sequential heating (12 vs 46 minutes).

Finally, continued device development has also led to increases in the overall maximum amount of power that can be delivered.[33,34] For RF-based devices, the maximum amount of RF current that can be delivered is dependent on both the generator output and the electrode surface area, as higher surface areas reduce the current density and therefore, adequate tissue heating around the electrode cannot be achieved. Whereas initial systems had maximum power outputs of less than 200 W, subsequent investigation suggests that higher current output and larger ablation zones can be achieved if higher-powered generators are coupled with larger-surface area electrodes. For example, Solazzo and colleagues[34] used a 500-KHz (1000 W) high-powered generator in an in vivo porcine model and achieved larger coagulation zones with a 4-cm tip cluster electrode (5.2 ± 0.8 cm) compared with a 2.5-cm cluster electrode (3.9 ± 0.3 cm). Similar gains in ablation size have been seen in higher-powered versions of microwave-based systems.[35]

Electrode Modification

Development of ablation applicators (electrodes for RF, antennae for microwave, and diffuser tips for laser-based systems) has contributed significantly to the ability to reliably achieve larger ablation zones. Several strategies to increase the amount of energy deposition and the overall ablation size have been balanced with the need for smaller-caliber electrodes to permit the continued use of these devices in a percutaneous and minimally invasive manner. These include the use of multiple electrodes simultaneously, either adjacent to each other or as part of an expandable device through a single introducer needle, the use of cooling systems to minimize tissue and electrode overheating, and the use of bipolar systems for RF ablation to increase tissue heating in the target zone.

Originally, simply lengthening the electrode tip increased coagulation in an asymmetric and preferentially longitudinal geometry. Use of a single electrode inserted multiple times to perform overlapping ablations requires significantly greater time and effort, making it impractical for routine use in a clinical setting. Therefore, the use of multiple electrodes simultaneously either in a pre-set configuration represents a significant step forward in increasing overall ablation size. Initial work with multiple electrodes demonstrated that placement of several monopolar electrodes in a clustered arrangement (no more than 1.5 cm apart) with simultaneous RF application could increase coagulation volume by more than 800% compared with a single electrode.[36] Subsequently, working to overcome the technical challenges of multiprobe application, multitined expandable RF electrodes have been developed.[37] These systems involve the deployment of a varying number of multiple thin, curved tines in the shape of an umbrella or more complex geometries from a central cannula.[38,39] This surmounts earlier difficulties by allowing easy placement of multiple probes to create large, reproducible volumes of necrosis. Leveen,[40] using a 12-hook array, was able to produce lesions measuring up to 3.5 cm in diameter in in vivo porcine liver by administering increasing amounts of RF energy from a 50-W RF generator for 10 minutes. More recently, Applebaum and colleagues[41] were able to achieve greater than 5 cm of coagulation in in vivo porcine liver using currently commercially available expandable electrodes with optimized stepped-extension and -power input algorithms.

Although most conventional RF systems use monopolar electrodes (where the current runs to remotely placed grounding pads placed on the patient's thighs to complete the circuit), several studies have reported results using bipolar arrays to increase the volume of coagulation created by RF application. In these systems, applied RF current runs from an active electrode to a second grounding electrode in place of a grounding pad. Heat is generated around both electrodes, creating elliptical lesions. McGahan and colleagues[42] used this method in ex vivo liver to induce necrosis of up to 4.0 cm in the long-axis diameter, but could only achieve 1.4 cm of necrosis in the short-axis diameter.[14] Although this increases the overall size of coagulation volume, the shape of necrosis is unsuitable for actual tumors, making the gains in coagulation less clinically significant. Desinger and colleagues[43] have described another bipolar array that contains both the active and return electrodes on the same 2-mm diameter probe. Lee and colleagues[44] used 2 multitined electrodes as active and return electrodes to increase coagulation during bipolar RF ablation. Finally, several studies have used a multipolar (more than 2) array of electrodes (multitined and single internally cooled) during RF ablation to achieve even greater volumes of coagulation.[45,46]

One of the limitations for RF-based systems has been overheating surrounding the active electrode, leading to tissue charring, rising impedance, and RF circuit interruption, ultimately limiting overall RF energy deposition. One successful strategy to address this has been the use of internal electrode cooling, whereby electrodes contain 2 hollow lumens that permit continuous internal cooling of the tip with a chilled perfusate, and the removal of warmed effluent to a collection unit outside of the body.[47] This reduces heating directly around the electrode, tissue charring, and rising impedance, allows greater RF energy deposition, and shifts the peak tissue temperature farther into the tumor, contributing to a broader depth of tissue heating from thermal conduction. In initial studies using cooling of 18-gauge single or clustered electrode needles with chilled 0°C saline perfusate, significant increases in RF energy deposition and ablation zone size were observed compared with conventional monopolar uncooled electrodes in ex vivo liver, with findings subsequently confirmed in in vivo large animal models and clinical studies.[29,47] Similar results were observed when chilled saline was infused in combination with expandable electrode systems (referred to as an "internally cooled wet electrode"), though infusion of fluid around the electrode is more difficult to control and makes the reproducibility of results more variable.[48] Most recently, several investigators have used alternative cooling agents (for example, argon or nitrogen gas) to achieve even greater cooling, and therefore larger zones of ablation, around the RF electrode tip.[49] As for RF-based systems, cooling of antennae shafts for microwave applicators has also been developed, which reduces shaft heating (and associated complications such as skin burns) while allowing increased power deposition through smaller-caliber antennae.

Although many of these technological advances have been developed independently of each other, they may often be used concurrently to achieve even larger ablation zones. Furthermore, while much of this work has been based on RF technology, specific techniques can be used for other thermal ablative therapies. For example, multiple electrodes and applicator cooling have been effectively applied in microwave-based systems as well.[50,51]

MODIFICATION OF THE BIOPHYSIOLOGIC ENVIRONMENT

Ablation research has traditionally focused on creating larger or more uniform reproducible zones of ablation through device and application development. However, device development is ultimately constrained by tumor and organ physiology. As such, many recent investigations have centered on altering underlying tumor physiology as a means to advance thermal ablation. Most studies to date have focused on the effects of tissue characteristics in the setting of temperature-based therapies in general (such as tissue perfusion and thermal conductivity), and system-specific characteristics, such as electrical conductivity for RF-based ablation.

Tissue Perfusion

The foremost factor limiting thermal ablation of tumors continues to be tissue blood flow, for which the effects are twofold. First, larger-diameter blood vessels with higher flow act as heat sinks, drawing away either heat (or cold) from the ablative area (**Fig. 2**).

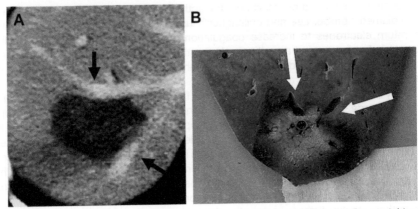

Fig. 2. Example of the heat-sink effect from large vessels on RF ablation. (*A*) An axial image from a delayed-phase contrast-enhanced CT scan demonstrates a focal area of hypoenhancement corresponding to an area previously treated with RF ablation. The medial aspect of the ablation zone is contained by 2 large hepatic veins (*arrows*); tissue heating was limited due to blood flow–mediated cooling. (*B*) Correlative gross pathologic cut sections of the liver demonstrate that the ablation zone is constrained along its medial edge by the 2 large hepatic veins (*arrows*).

For example, in a study in an in vivo porcine model, Monsky and colleagues[52] examined the effect of hepatic vessel diameter on RF ablation outcome. Using computed tomography (CT) and histopathologic analysis, more complete thermal heating and a reduced heat-sink effect was identified when hepatic vessels within the heating zone were less than 3 mm in diameter. In contrast, vessels greater than 3 mm in diameter had higher patency rates, less endothelial injury, and greater viability of surrounding hepatocytes after RF ablation. This strong predictive nature of hepatic blood flow on the extent of RF induced coagulation has been confirmed in multiple studies where increased coagulation volumes have been obtained when hepatic blood flow is decreased, either by balloon or coil embolization or the Pringle maneuver.[53] The second effect of tissue vasculature is a result of perfusion-mediated tissue cooling (capillary vascular flow) that also functions as a heat sink. By drawing heat from the treatment zone, this effect reduces the volume of tissue that receives the required minimal thermal dose for coagulation. Along with the use of mechanical occlusion, several studies have also used pharmacologic alteration of tissue perfusion to reduce these effects. Goldberg and colleagues[54] modulated hepatic blood flow using intra-arterial vasopressin and high-dose halothane in conjunction with RF ablation in in vivo porcine liver. Arsenic trioxide, which has recently received increasing attention as a novel antineoplastic agent,[49,55] has been shown to preferentially decrease tumor blood flow and significantly increase RF-induced coagulation in a renal tumor model.[49] More recently, promising antiangiogenic therapies, such as sorafenib, are also starting to be studied as combination therapies with ablation, with similar encouraging effects in animals[56] leading to the initiation of clinical trials.

Thermal Conductivity

Initial clinical studies using RF ablation for hepatocellular carcinoma in the setting of underlying cirrhosis noted an "oven" effect (ie, increased heating efficacy for tumors surrounded by cirrhotic liver or fat, such as exophytic renal cell carcinomas), or altered thermal transmission at the junction of tumor tissue and surrounding tissue.[3] Subsequent experimental studies in ex vivo agar phantoms and bovine liver have confirmed the effects of varying tumor and surrounding tissue thermal conductivity on effective heat transmission during RF ablation, and have further demonstrated the role of "optimal" thermal conductivity characteristics on ablation outcomes.[16,57] For example, very poor tumor thermal conductivity limits heat transmission centrifugally away from the electrode with marked heating in the central portion of the tumor, and limited, potentially incomplete heating in peripheral portions of the tumor. By contrast, increased thermal conductivity (such as in cystic lesions) results in fast heat transmission (ie, heat dissipation), with potentially incomplete and heterogeneous tumor heating. Furthermore, in recent agar phantom and computer modeling studies, Liu and colleagues[57] demonstrated that differences in thermal conductivity between the tumor and surrounding background tissue (specifically, decreased thermal conductivity from increased fat content of surrounding tissue) results in increased temperatures at the tumor margin. However, heating was limited in the surrounding medium, making a 1-cm "ablative" margin difficult to achieve. An understanding of the role of thermal conductivity, and tissue- and tumor-specific characteristics, on tissue heating may be useful when trying to predict ablation outcome in varying clinical settings (eg, in exophytic renal cell carcinomas surrounded by perirenal fat, lung tumors surrounded by aerated normal parenchyma, or osseous metastases surrounded by cortical bone).[16]

Electrical Conductivity

Local electrical conductivity is a tissue characteristic that specifically influences energy deposition in RF-based systems. RF-induced tissue heating, generated by resistive heating from ionic agitation, is strongly dependent on the local electrical conductivity. To this end, the effect of local electrical conductivity on RF-induced tissue heating can be broadly divided into 2 categories. First, altering the electrical environment immediately around the RF electrode with ionic agents can increase electrical conductivity before or during RF ablation. The increase in conductivity allows greater energy deposition and, therefore, increased coagulation volume.[4,58] Saline may also be of benefit when attempting to ablate cavitary lesions that might not otherwise contain a sufficient current path. In general, small volumes of highly concentrated sodium ions are injected in and around the ablation site to maximize local heating effects, findings observed in both experimental and clinical studies and subsequently incorporated into electrode development.[59] However, it should be noted that saline infusion is not always a predictable process, as fluid can migrate to unintended locations and cause complications if not used properly.[60]

Second, differences in electrical conductivity between the tumor and surrounding background organ can affect tissue heating at the tumor margin. Several studies have demonstrated increases in tissue heating at the tumor-organ interface when the surrounding medium is characterized by reduced lower electrical conductivity.[61] In certain clinical settings, such as treating focal tumors in either lung or bone, marked differences in electrical conductivity may result in variable heating at the tumor/organ interface, and indeed limit heating in the surrounding organ, and may make obtaining a 1.0-cm ablative margin difficult.

Finally, electrical conductivity must be taken into account when using techniques such as hydrodissection to protect adjacent organs. Nonionic fluids can be used to protect tissues adjacent to the ablation zone (such as diaphragm or bowel) from thermal injury. For this application, fluids with low ion content, such as 5% dextrose in water (D5W), should be used because they have been proven to electrically force

RF current away from the protected organ, decrease the size and incidence of burns on the diaphragm and bowel, and reduce pain scores in patients treated with D5W when compared with ionic solutions, such as saline.[31,32] Ionic solutions such as 0.9% saline should not be used for hydrodissection because, as noted, they actually increase RF current flow.[62]

COMBINING THERMAL ABLATION WITH ADJUVANT THERAPIES

While substantial efforts have been made in modifying ablation systems and the biologic environment to improve the clinical utility of percutaneous ablation, limitations in clinical efficacy persist. For example, with further long-term follow-up of patients undergoing ablation therapy, there has been an increased incidence of detection of progressive local tumor growth for all tumor types and sizes despite initial indications of adequate therapy, suggesting that there are residual foci of viable, untreated disease in a substantial, but unknown number of cases.[3] The ability to achieve complete and uniform eradication of all malignant cells remains a key barrier to clinical success, and therefore strategies that can increase the completeness of RF tumor destruction, even for small lesions, are needed.

Investigators have sought to improve results by combining thermal ablation with adjuvant therapies such as radiation and chemotherapy.[63,64] At present, thermal ablation only takes advantage of temperatures that are sufficient by themselves to induce coagulation necrosis (>50°C). Yet, based on the exponential decrease in RF tissue heating, there is a steep thermal gradient in tissues surrounding an RF electrode. Hence, there is substantial flattening of the curve below 50°C, with a much larger tissue volume encompassed by the 45°C isotherm. Modeling studies demonstrate that were the threshold for cell death to be decreased by as few as 5°C, tumor coagulation could be increased up to 1.5 cm (up to a 59% increase in spherical volume of the ablation zone).[61] Therefore, target tumors can be conceptually divided into 3 zones: (1) a central area, predominantly treated by thermal ablation, which undergoes heat-induced coagulation necrosis, (2) a peripheral rim, which undergoes reversible changes from sublethal hyperthermia, and (3) surrounding tumor or normal tissue that is unaffected by focal ablation, though still exposed to adjuvant systemic therapies.

Several studies have demonstrated that tumor death can be enhanced when combining RF thermal therapy with adjuvant chemo- or radiosensitizers. The goal of this combined approach is to increase tumor destruction occurring within the sizable peripheral zone of sublethal temperatures (ie, largely reversible cell damage induced by mildly elevating tissue temperatures to 41°C–45°C) surrounding the heat-induced coagulation.[63] Improved tumor cytotoxicity is also likely to reduce the local recurrence rate at the treatment site. Although there is high-temperature heating throughout the zone of RF ablation, heterogeneity of thermal diffusion (especially in the presence of vascularity) retards uniform and complete ablation.[65] Because local control requires complete tumor destruction, ablation may be inadequate even if large zones of ablation that encompass the entire tumor are created. By killing tumor cells at lower temperatures, this combined paradigm will not only increase necrosis volume but may also create a more complete area of tumor destruction by filling in untreated gaps within the ablation zone.[66] Combined treatment also has the potential to achieve equivalent tumor destruction with a concomitant reduction of the duration or course of therapy (a process which currently takes hours to treat larger tumors, with many protocols requiring repeat sessions). A reduction in the time required to completely ablate a given tumor volume would permit patients with larger or greater numbers of tumors to be treated. Shorter heating time could also potentially improve the quality of life of patients by reducing the number of visits and the substantial costs of prolonged procedures that require image guidance.

Combining Thermal Ablation with Adjuvant Chemotherapy

Several investigators have combined thermal ablation with adjuvant chemotherapy, mostly using RF and doxorubicin-based regimens.[63,67,68] Given the potential synergy of combining therapies, an initial study administered RF ablation in conjunction with percutaneous intratumoral injection of injected free doxorubicin in a rat breast adeno-carcinoma model, and demonstrated increases in mean tumor necrosis diameter with combination doxorubicin and RF therapy (11.4 mm) compared with RF alone (6.7 mm).[69] However, as initial image-guided direct intratumoral injection strategies have encountered many difficulties in clinical practice such as nonuniform drug diffu-sion and limited operator control on drug distribution, subsequent studies have combined RF ablation with doxorubicin encapsulated within a liposome.[66,70] Lipo-some particles are completely biocompatible, cause very little toxic or antigenic reac-tion, and are biologically inert. Water-soluble drugs can be trapped in the inner aqueous compartment, whereas lipophilic compounds may be incorporated into the liposomal lipid membrane. In addition, incorporation of polyethyleneglycol surface modifications minimizes plasma protein absorption on liposome surfaces and subse-quent recognition and uptake of liposomes by the reticuloendothelial system, which further reduces systemic phagocytosis and results in prolonged circulation time, selective agent delivery through the leaky tumor endothelium (an enhanced perme-ability and retention effect), and reduced toxicity profiles.[71,72] As a result, this doxoru-bicin-containing formulation has become widely accepted for clinical practice.[73–75]

Several studies have combined RF ablation with a commercially available form of liposomal doxorubicin (Doxil). Experiments in a rat breast adenocarcinoma have demonstrated significant increases in mean tumor coagulation diameter from combi-nation RF/Doxil therapy (13.1 mm) compared with RF alone (6.7 mm).[76] Of note, RF ablation combined with adjuvant empty liposomes also increased coagulation over RF alone but less than RF/Doxil.[76] Increases in tumor necrosis with combination RF/Doxil were subsequently confirmed in larger animal tumor models and a pilot clin-ical study.[66,70] For example, in a large animal canine subcutaneous sarcoma model, combination therapy increased mean tumor coagulation diameter from 23 mm with RF alone to 37 mm with RF/Doxil, representing an increase of 212% in necrosis volume, with most of the gain occurring in the larger peripheral periablative zone.[70] In addition, D'Ippolito and colleagues[77] reported increases in animal end-point survival for rat R3230 adenocarcinoma tumors treated with combined RF/intravenous liposomal chemotherapy (28 days) compared with either RF or intravenous liposomal chemotherapy alone (18 days each).

In a pilot clinical study combining RF ablation (internally cooled electrode) with adju-vant liposomal doxorubicin, 10 patients with 18 intrahepatic tumors were randomized to receive either liposomal doxorubicin (20 mg Doxil) 24 hours before RF ablation or RF ablation alone (mean tumor size undergoing ablation was 4.0 ± 1.8 cm).[66] Whereas no difference in the amount of tumor destruction was seen between groups immediately following RF, at 2 to 4 weeks, patients receiving liposomal doxorubicin had an increase in tumor destruction of 24% to 342% volumetric increase (median = 32%) compared with a decrease of 76% to 88% for treatment with RF alone (a finding concordant with prior observations). Several additional and clinically beneficial find-ings were also observed only in the combination therapy group, including increased diameter of the treatment effect for multiple tumor types, improved completeness of tumor destruction particularly adjacent to intratumoral vessels, and increased treatment effect including the peritumoral liver parenchyma (suggesting a contribution to achieving an adequate ablative margin).

The processes governing increases in tumor destruction with combined RF/intravenous liposomal doxorubicin are likely multifactorial, and reflect both increased intratumoral drug delivery and combined 2-hit cytotoxic effects of exposure to nonlethal low-level hyperthermia in periablational tumor and adjuvant chemotherapy. Noncoagulative hyperthermia increases intratumoral drug accumulation through increases in intratumoral blood flow and microvascular permeability, likely as a result of endothelial injury and increases in vascular endothelial pore size. Studies in both small and large animal models have demonstrated up to a 5.6-fold increase in intratumoral doxorubicin accumulation following RF ablation, adding that (1) the greatest amount of intratumoral doxorubicin occurs in the zone immediately peripheral to the central RF area, and (2) smaller amounts of doxorubicin were found in the central RF-coagulated area, suggesting drug deposition in areas with residual, patent vasculature.[52] These findings help explain why liposomal doxorubicin is likely to be complementary to RF ablation. The majority of the liposomes was concentrated in a zone immediately peripheral to the area coagulated by RF heating and within the region where nonlethal hyperthermia and increased destruction is observed.[78] In addition, the patchy penetration of liposomes into the zone of coagulation implies infiltration of chemotherapy into the coagulated focus (possibly through residual patent vessels) that may improve the completeness of tumor destruction. Finally, several liposomal formulations are available that have chemical structures designed to release their contents at specific hyperthermic temperatures (42°C–45°C), further increasing the specificity of targeting periablational tumors.[79]

Separate from increased intratumoral drug accumulation, several mechanisms for increased tumor destruction have also been identified, most notably increased cell stress (in part due to upregulation of nitrative and oxidative pathways) leading to apoptosis.[80] Recently, Solazzo and colleagues[80] performed immunohistochemical staining of rat breast tumors treated with RF ablation with and without adjuvant Doxil for markers of cellular stress. In the periablational rim surrounding the ablation zone, combination RF/Doxil increased markers of DNA breakage and oxidative and nitrative stress early ($\sim$4 hours) after RF ablation, with subsequent colocalization staining for cleaved caspase-3 (a marker for apoptosis), suggesting that these areas later underwent apoptosis. N-Acetylcysteine was also administered in some animals, and reductions in both cellular stress pathways and apoptosis confirmed the causal relationship between the 2 processes. In addition, increased heat-shock protein production in a concentric ring of still-viable tumor surrounding the ablation zone, and immediately peripheral to the rim of apoptosis, was also observed.

This greater understanding of underlying mechanisms has led to successful investigations into the use of additional adjuvant chemotherapies that specifically target cellular stress pathways. In a recent study, Yang and colleagues[81] combined RF ablation with intravenous liposomal paclitaxel, an agent with known proapoptotic and anti–heat-shock protein effects, in subcutaneous rat breast adenocarcinoma tumors. Combination RF-paclitaxel increased tumor coagulation and animal survival compared with RF alone, with even greater gains observed for RF-paclitaxel-Doxil. Of note, immunohistochemistry demonstrated reduced heat-shock protein expression and increased apoptosis for treatment combinations that included paclitaxel. Most recently, combining RF ablation with intravenous liposomal quercetin (a flavonoid agent with known anti–heat-shock protein effects) also reduced heat-shock protein expression and increased tumor coagulation and survival.[82] Based on these results, it is becoming clear that judicious selection of the type of chemotherapy combined with thermal therapy is necessary to potentiate and optimize the tumoricidal effects occurring in the peripheral zone of hyperthermia created by RF heating, along with tailored regimens that are tumor and organ type specific.

Finally, given the effects of RF on increasing intratumoral drug delivery, the use of short courses of RF to concentrate liposomally delivered drugs could potentially expand the clinical use of this and other chemotherapeutic agents that have previously lacked efficacy due to their inability to achieve sufficient intratumoral drug concentrations. In addition, selective intratumoral deposition of high drug concentrations could potentially allow an overall reduction of drug dosage,[76] thereby reducing the potential for systemic toxicity while maintaining delivery of high doses to the tumor target. Thus, liposomal delivery into ablated tumors has the unique potential to act as a focal targeting mechanism to guide the deposition of liposome encapsulated agents.[76,83]

Combining Thermal Ablation with Adjuvant Radiation

Several studies have reported early investigation into combination RF ablation and radiation therapy, with promising results.[64,84] There are known synergistic effects of combined external-beam radiation therapy and low-temperature hyperthermia.[85] Experimental animal studies have demonstrated increased tumor necrosis, reduced tumor growth, and improved animal survival with combined external beam radiation and RF ablation when compared with either therapy alone.[64,86] For example, in a rat breast adenocarcinoma model, Horkan and colleagues[64] demonstrated significantly longer mean end-point survival for animals treated with combination RF ablation and 20-Gy external beam radiation (94 days) compared with either radiation (40 days) or RF ablation (20 days) alone. Preliminary clinical studies in primary lung malignancies confirm the synergistic effects of these therapies. Potential causes for the synergy include the sensitization of the tumor to subsequent radiation, due to the increased oxygenation resulting from hyperthermia-induced increased blood flow to the tumor.[87] Another possible mechanism, which has been seen in animal tumor models, is an inhibition of radiation-induced repair and recovery and increased free radical formation.[80] Future work is needed to identify the optimal temperature for ablation and optimal radiation dose, as well as the most effective method of administering radiation therapy (external-beam radiation therapy, brachytherapy, or yttrium microspheres), on an organ-by-organ basis.

IMPROVING IMAGE GUIDANCE AND TUMOR TARGETING

Thermal ablation is commonly performed with a percutaneous approach using imaging guidance with a single or combination of modalities (CT, ultrasound, or magnetic resonance imaging [MRI]). A successful ablation is contingent on the operator's ability to visualize the tumor, position the electrode within the target, and accurately evaluate the treatment zone on ablation completion. Several significant challenges to performing a successful ablation exist at each of these steps. For example, diagnostic imaging studies are often obtained with modalities that are separate from the modality being used for treatment (for example, diagnostic MRI and ablation being performed with CT or ultrasound), positional variations between diagnostic and treatment imaging preclude an exact overlay of different imaging studies, and target tumors are often highly variable in their imaging appearance in a modality-specific manner (for example, a focal hepatocellular carcinoma may be clearly visible on MRI, barely visible on ultrasonography, and invisible with noncontrast enhanced CT). Electrode positioning often requires traversing a narrow course or window in a 3-dimensional trajectory when only 2-dimensional real-time imaging is available, often when the target is moving from respiratory motion. Finally, correlating the immediate postprocedure imaging to prior diagnostic imaging to determine adequacy of treatment, especially at the tumor margin, can often be difficult. All of these factors make the treatment of some lesions extremely technically challenging.[88]

Several technologies are being developed to address some of these difficulties.[88] Image-fusion software is now becoming commercially available to allow image overlay of 2 different imaging modalities for diagnostic interpretation. Multimodality image fusion for procedural guidance takes this further by pairing an existing data set from a prior diagnostic study to the real-time modality being used for the procedure. CT-ultrasound fusion systems often use a sensor in the ultrasound transducer and initial landmark localization to fuse a prior CT scan (which allows multiplanar reconstruction from the CT data set) with real-time ultrasound images (**Fig. 3**). Finally, needle-tracking systems are also being developed using either electromagnetic (EM) or optical (infrared-based) tracking technology.[89] In these systems, the needle tip is identified and localized in 3-dimensional space and the needle trajectory overlays existing imaging. EM-based devices use a small field generator to create a rapidly changing magnetic field, in which a sensor coil in the needle tip creates an electrical current, allowing localization within 3-dimensional space. Several of these devices have been tested for simple procedures such as joint injection or biopsy, and can likely be applied to ablative procedures as well.[90,91]

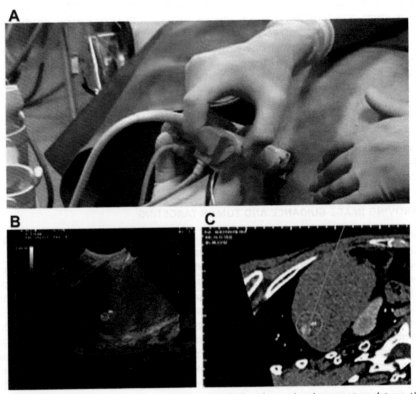

Fig. 3. Use of image-guided CT-US fusion to assist in electrode placement and targeting during RF ablation. (*A*) Example of US guidance for tumor targeting and electrode placement. (*B, C*) Real-time US imaging is acquired and merged with data from an existing CT scan, allowing identification of the target lesion for electrode placement and ablation.

STRATEGIES FOR TRANSLATING BASIC SCIENCE RESEARCH INTO CLINICAL PRACTICE

Since its original use for primary hepatic tumors, there have been several advances in the clinical effectiveness and application of thermal ablation, including successful expansion of its use for larger tumors and in varying organs. However, as the need for continued improvement in clinical ablation efficacy persists, research continues to improve existing techniques and develop additional technologies. A critical component of this is the successful translation of investigative laboratory research into clinical practice. To this end, effective ablation research of new devices and techniques is contingent on the achievement of several objectives: (1) appropriate characterization in a laboratory setting; (2) refinement and optimization in a laboratory setting using appropriate models that reflect real clinical circumstances; and (3) successful application in appropriate clinical cases and patients. The successful completion of these objectives requires the rational use of both small animal tumor models combined with larger nontumor animal models and the incorporation of computer modeling systems that can improve treatment characterization and predictability.

Effectively Incorporating Animal Models into Thermal Ablation Research

Successful translation of experimental studies to clinical practice requires an integrated use of various ex vivo and in vivo models. While initial thermal ablative device characterization is commonly performed in ex vivo models (for example, porcine or bovine liver), direct extrapolation of results to clinical situations is limited because these models do not take into account significant underlying tumor and organ physiology. For example, hepatic blood flow has a marked negative effect on ablative heating and is not accurately represented in ex vivo models. In an original study using an internally cooled cluster electrode, RF ablation induced 4.7 cm of coagulation in ex vivo liver compared with 3.1 cm in in vivo porcine liver.[29,47] Therefore, many studies use an in vivo large nontumor animal model (most commonly, normal pig) for testing experimental devices for liver ablation. This model is useful, as it has a similarly sized organ anatomy to humans and therefore allows appropriate comparison testing of actual clinical devices in a preclinical setting. However, one main disadvantage is that it does not approximate actual tumor biology, including known differences in tissue heating and biology between tumor and normal hepatic parenchyma.

More recently, small animal tumor models have also been increasingly used in ablation research, especially with the use of adjuvant therapies, when needing to understand the interaction of tumor and ablative biophysiology, and when the primary question being investigated is specific to tumor biology. Advantages of these models include closer approximation of actual tumor type–specific biology (compared with in vivo normal porcine liver, for example), as represented by implanting human-based tumor cell lines into immunosuppressed or knockout mice. Additional benefits are low cost and easy availability, and the potential to perform larger-volume characterization studies. Several investigators have successfully used these models to investigate mechanisms of action in combination ablation/chemotherapy studies.

Disadvantages of smaller models are that they have limited utility in device development given the small size of tumors (most experimental ablations in these models use a scaled-down model of an ablative device, such as a smaller caliber and electrode length). Several larger animal tumor models exist, including VX2 adenocarcinoma implantable in multiple organ sites in rabbits, and canine venereal sarcoma (also known as transmissible venereal tumor) in dogs. However, limitations with these larger models include persistent tumor size limitations in rabbits, prohibitive time and cost requirements for canine models, and limited biologic correlation to human tumors.

Recently, Aravalli and colleagues[92] published a comprehensive review of currently available and commonly used animals in thermal ablation research. Ultimately, successful and comprehensive thermal ablation research involves an integrated use of available models. Effective research study design and use of resources will be based on identifying the specific question being asked, and then tailoring the choice of animal or computer model to most effectively arrive at the answer.

The Role of Computer Modeling in Thermal Ablation Research

One of the main limitations of using in vivo animal models alone in thermal ablation research is that given the inherent variability within in vivo models, complete characterization of the multifactorial energy-tissue interactions in thermal ablation is too complex for initial direct clinical interrogation. Several investigators have developed computer simulation models of thermal ablation that use tumor- and tissue-specific measurements of key variables of the Bioheat equation to calculate multiple points of tissue heating. These models are able to simulate percutaneous treatment of focal tumors by predicting tissue heating patterns for various clinical situations.[16,93,94] Existing experimental approaches to modeling single variables or scenarios have been limited in completely predicting thermal ablation given the heterogeneous target clinical population, the complex number of variable tissue parameters, the time-consuming approach of single-variable interrogation, and the heterogeneity of tumor and background organ biology and physiology.

More recent investigation has also evolved to incorporate both single and 2-compartment finite-element computer modeling as a more realistic and clinically relevant simulation for improving the understanding of tissue heating patterns and tissue-energy interactions.[16,94] Advantages of computer modeling include the ability to interrogate individual parameters in isolation or in combination, clarify their potential influence on energy deposition and tissue heating over a wide and clinically relevant physiologic range, separate out the specific environments in which certain variables demonstrate a more dominant effect, and characterize the effects of differences in tissue and tumor characteristics, especially at the tumor margin. This strategy may be helpful in better understanding heating for specific tumor and organ situations, and therefore improving RF predictability. Nevertheless, although preliminary results with computer modeling have been useful, predictive accuracy and clinical validation of their results are needed. Successful validation with subsequent translation to clinically relevant large animal models will establish greater predictability of thermal coagulation, and set the stage for rapid clinical translation and subsequent implementation.

Finally, there is a recent report of using computer modeling to characterize and predict intratumoral drug deposition when RF ablation was combined with adjuvant doxorubicin, either in a free form or encapsulated within thermosensitive liposomes. Gasselhuber and colleagues,[95] using spatial and temporal tissue heating and perfusion to create a multicompartment pharmacokinetic model to predict drug release and intratumoral drug concentrations, reported good correlation of the model findings to in vivo results. This study underscores the potential role of computer modeling in improving treatment predictability in all aspects of thermal ablation research.

SUMMARY

As thermal ablation is being used for an increasing number of tumor types and in varied organ settings, a thorough understanding of the basic principles and recent advances in thermal ablation is a necessary prerequisite to their effective clinical use. Several successful strategies have been used to improve thermal ablation efficacy involving technological advancements in ablation devices, including electrode and navigation system developments and modifications of tissue and tumor environment. Recent studies have used computer modeling to improve the understanding of tissue heating patterns. Finally, thermal ablation has been successfully combined with adjuvant chemotherapy and radiation, and future investigation will explore tailoring specific adjuvant therapies based on a mechanistic rationale.

REFERENCES

1. Gervais DA, McGovern FJ, Arellano RS, et al. Renal cell carcinoma: clinical experience and technical success with radio-frequency ablation of 42 tumors. Radiology 2003;226:417–24.
2. Kurup AN, Callstrom MR. Ablation of skeletal metastases: current status. J Vasc Interv Radiol 2010;21:S242–50.
3. Livraghi T, Meloni F, Goldberg SN, et al. Hepatocellular carcinoma: radiofrequency ablation of medium and large lesions. Radiology 2000;214:761–8.
4. Solbiati L, Livraghi T, Goldberg SN, et al. Percutaneous radiofrequency ablation of hepatic metastases from colorectal cancer: long term results in 117 patients. Radiology 2001;221:159–66.
5. Venkatesan AM, Locklin J, Dupuy DE, et al. Percutaneous ablation of adrenal tumors. Tech Vasc Interv Radiol 2010;13:89–99.
6. Zemlyak A, Moore WH, Bilfinger TV. Comparison of survival after sublobar resections and ablative therapies for stage I non-small cell lung cancer. J Am Coll Surg 2010;211:68–72.
7. McWilliams JP, Yamamoto S, Raman SS, et al. Percutaneous ablation of hepatocellular carcinoma: current status. J Vasc Interv Radiol 2010;21:S204–13.
8. Dodd GD 3rd, Soulen MC, Kane RA, et al. Minimally invasive treatment of malignant hepatic tumors: at the threshold of a major breakthrough. Radiographics 2000;20:9–27.
9. Shimada K, Sakamoto Y, Esaki M, et al. Role of the width of the surgical margin in a hepatectomy for small hepatocellular carcinomas eligible for percutaneous local ablative therapy. Am J Surg 2008;195:775–81.
10. Gervais DA, McGovern FJ, Arellano RS, et al. Radiofrequency ablation of renal cell carcinoma: part 1, Indications, results, and role in patient management over a 6-year period and ablation of 100 tumors. AJR Am J Roentgenol 2005; 185:64–71.
11. Lencioni R, Cioni D, Crocetti L, et al. Early-stage hepatocellular carcinoma in patients with cirrhosis: long-term results of percutaneous image-guided radiofrequency ablation. Radiology 2005;234:961–7.
12. Lencioni R, Crocetti L, Cioni R, et al. Response to radiofrequency ablation of pulmonary tumours: a prospective, intention-to-treat, multicentre clinical trial (the RAPTURE study). Lancet Oncol 2008;9:621–8.
13. Dodd GD 3rd, Frank MS, Aribandi M, et al. Radiofrequency thermal ablation: computer analysis of the size of the thermal injury created by overlapping ablations. AJR Am J Roentgenol 2001;177:777–82.
14. Goldberg SN, Grassi CJ, Cardella JF, et al. Image-guided tumor ablation: standardization of terminology and reporting criteria. J Vasc Interv Radiol 2009;20: S377–90.
15. Schramm W, Yang D, Haemmerich D. Contribution of direct heating, thermal conduction and perfusion during radiofrequency and microwave ablation. Conf Proc IEEE Eng Med Biol Soc 2006;1:5013–6.

16. Ahmed M, Liu Z, Humphries S, et al. Computer modeling of the combined effects of perfusion, electrical conductivity, and thermal conductivity on tissue heating patterns in radiofrequency tumor ablation. Int J Hyperthermia 2008;24: 577–88.

17. Seegenschmiedt M, Brady L, Sauer R. Interstitial thermoradiotherapy: review on technical and clinical aspects. Am J Clin Oncol 1990;13:352–63.

18. Trembley B, Ryan T, Strohbehn J. Interstitial hyperthermia: physics, biology, and clinical aspects. Hyperthermia and Oncology, vol. 3. Utrecht (The Netherlands): VSP; 1992. p. 11–98.

19. Larson T, Bostwick D, Corcia A. Temperature-correlated histopathologic changes following microwave thermoablation of obstructive tissues in patients with benign prostatic hyperplasia. Urology 1996;47:463–9.

20. Zevas N, Kuwayama A. Pathologic analysis of experimental thermal lesions: comparison of induction heating and radiofrequency electrocoagulation. J Neurosurg 1972;37:418–22.

21. Goldberg SN, Gazelle GS, Compton CC, et al. Treatment of intrahepatic malignancy with radiofrequency ablation: radiologic-pathologic correlation. Cancer 2000;88:2452–63.

22. Goldberg SN, Gazelle GS, Halpern EF, et al. Radiofrequency tissue ablation: importance of local temperature along the electrode tip exposure in determining lesion shape and size. Acad Radiol 1996;3:212–8.

23. Mertyna P, Dewhirst MW, Halpern E, et al. Radiofrequency ablation: the effect of distance and baseline temperature on thermal dose required for coagulation. Int J Hyperthermia 2008;24:550–9.

24. Mertyna P, Hines-Peralta A, Liu ZJ, et al. Radiofrequency ablation: variability in heat sensitivity in tumors and tissues. J Vasc Interv Radiol 2007;18:647–54.

25. Goldberg SN, Gazelle GS, Dawson SL, et al. Tissue ablation with radiofrequency: effect of probe size, gauge, duration, and temperature on lesion volume. Acad Radiol 1995;2:399–404.

26. Pennes H. Analysis of tissue and arterial blood temperatures in the resting human forearm. J Appl Physiol 1948;1:93–122.

27. Goldberg SN, Gazelle GS, Mueller PR. Thermal ablation therapy for focal malignancy: a unified approach to underlying principles, techniques, and diagnostic imaging guidance. AJR Am J Roentgenol 2000;174:323–31.

28. Goldberg SN, Stein M, Gazelle GS, et al. Percutaneous radiofrequency tissue ablation: optimization of pulsed-RF technique to increase coagulation necrosis. J Vasc Interv Radiol 1999;10:907–16.

29. Goldberg SN, Solbiati L, Hahn PF, et al. Large-volume tissue ablation with radio frequency by using a clustered, internally cooled electrode technique: laboratory and clinical experience in liver metastases. Radiology 1998;209:371–9.

30. Gulesserian T, Mahnken AH, Schernthaner R, et al. Comparison of expandable electrodes in percutaneous radiofrequency ablation of renal cell carcinoma. Eur J Radiol 2006;59:133–9.

31. Brace CL, Sampson LA, Hinshaw JL, et al. Radiofrequency ablation: simultaneous application of multiple electrodes via switching creates larger, more confluent ablations than sequential application in a large animal model. J Vasc Interv Radiol 2009;20:118–24.

32. Laeseke PF, Sampson LA, Haemmerich D, et al. Multiple-electrode radiofrequency ablation creates confluent areas of necrosis: in vivo porcine liver results. Radiology 2006;241:116–24.

33. Brace CL, Laeseke PF, Sampson LA, et al. Radiofrequency ablation with a high-power generator: device efficacy in an in vivo porcine liver model. Int J Hyperthermia 2007;23:387–94.

34. Solazzo SA, Ahmed M, Liu Z, et al. High-power generator for radiofrequency ablation: larger electrodes and pulsing algorithms in bovine ex vivo and porcine in vivo settings. Radiology 2007;242:743–50.

35. Laeseke PF, Lee FT Jr, Sampson LA, et al. Microwave ablation versus radiofrequency ablation in the kidney: high-power triaxial antennas create larger ablation zones than similarly sized internally cooled electrodes. J Vasc Interv Radiol 2009; 20:1224–9.

36. Goldberg SN, Gazelle GS, Dawson SL, et al. Radiofrequency tissue ablation using multiprobe arrays: greater tissue destruction than multiple probes operating alone. Acad Radiol 1995;2:670–4.

37. Bangard C, Rosgen S, Wahba R, et al. Large-volume multi-tined expandable RF ablation in pig livers: comparison of 2D and volumetric measurements of the ablation zone. Eur Radiol 2010;20:1073–8.

38. Rossi S, Buscarini E, Garbagnati F. Percutaneous treatment of small hepatic tumors by an expandable RF needle electrode. AJR Am J Roentgenol 1998; 170:1015–22.

39. Siperstein AE, Rogers SJ, Hansen PD, et al. Laparoscopic thermal ablation of hepatic neuroendocrine tumor metastases. Surgery 1997;122:1147–55.

40. Leveen RF. Laser hyperthermia and radiofrequency ablation of hepatic lesions. Semin Intervent Radiol 1997;12:313–24.

41. Appelbaum L, Sosna J, Pearson R, et al. Algorithm optimization for multitined radiofrequency ablation: comparative study in ex vivo and in vivo bovine liver. Radiology 2010;254:430–40.

42. McGahan JP, Gu WZ, Brock JM, et al. Hepatic ablation using bipolar radiofrequency electrocautery. Acad Radiol 1996;3(5):418–22.

43. Desinger K, Stein T, Muller G, et al. Interstitial bipolar RF-thermotherapy (REITT) therapy by planning by computer simulation and MRI-monitoring—a new concept for minimally invasive procedures. Proc SPIE 1999;3249:147–60.

44. Lee JM, Han JK, Kim SH, et al. Bipolar radiofrequency ablation using wet-cooled electrodes: an in vitro experimental study in bovine liver. AJR Am J Roentgenol 2005;184:391–7.

45. Seror O, N'Kontchou G, Ibraheem M, et al. Large (>or = 5.0-cm) HCCs: multipolar RF ablation with three internally cooled bipolar electrodes—initial experience in 26 patients. Radiology 2008;248:288–96.

46. Lee JM, Han JK, Kim HC, et al. Multiple-electrode radiofrequency ablation of in vivo porcine liver: comparative studies of consecutive monopolar, switching monopolar versus multipolar modes. Invest Radiol 2007;42:676–83.

47. Goldberg SN, Gazelle GS, Solbiati L, et al. Radiofrequency tissue ablation: increased lesion diameter with a perfusion electrode. Acad Radiol 1996;3:636–44.

48. Cha J, Choi D, Lee MW, et al. Radiofrequency ablation zones in ex vivo bovine and in vivo porcine livers: comparison of the use of internally cooled electrodes and internally cooled wet electrodes. Cardiovasc Intervent Radiol 2009;32: 1235–40.

49. Hines-Peralta A, Hollander CY, Solazzo S, et al. Hybrid radiofrequency and cryoablation device: preliminary results in an animal model. J Vasc Interv Radiol 2004;15:1111–20.

50. Cheng Z, Xiao Q, Wang Y, et al. 915MHz microwave ablation with implanted internal cooled-shaft antenna: initial experimental study in in vivo porcine livers. Eur J Radiol 2010. [Epub ahead of print].
51. He N, Wang W, Ji Z, et al. Microwave ablation: an experimental comparative study on internally cooled antenna versus non-internally cooled antenna in liver models. Acad Radiol 2010;17:894–9.
52. Monsky WL, Kruskal JB, Lukyanov AN, et al. Radio-frequency ablation increases intratumoral liposomal doxorubicin accumulation in a rat breast tumor model. Radiology 2002;224:823–9.
53. Patterson EJ, Scudamore CH, Owen DA, et al. Radiofrequency ablation of porcine liver in vivo: effects of blood flow and treatment time on lesion size. Ann Surg 1998;227:559–65.
54. Goldberg SN, Hahn PF, Halpern EF, et al. Radiofrequency tissue ablation: effect of pharmacologic modulation of blood flow on coagulation diameter. Radiology 1998;209:761–9.
55. Hines-Peralta A, Sukhatme V, Regan M, et al. Improved tumor destruction with arsenic trioxide and radiofrequency ablation in three animal models. Radiology 2006;240:82–9.
56. Hakime A, Hines-Peralta A, Peddi H, et al. Combination of radiofrequency ablation with antiangiogenic therapy for tumor ablation efficacy: study in mice. Radiology 2007;244:464–70.
57. Liu Z, Ahmed M, Weinstein Y, et al. Characterization of the RF ablation-induced 'oven effect': the importance of background tissue thermal conductivity on tissue heating. Int J Hyperthermia 2006;22:327–42.
58. Aube C, Schmidt D, Brieger J, et al. Influence of NaCl concentrations on coagulation, temperature, and electrical conductivity using a perfusion radiofrequency ablation system: an ex vivo experimental study. Cardiovasc Intervent Radiol 2007;30:92–7.
59. Miao Y, Ni Y, Yu J, et al. A comparative study on validation of a novel cooled-wet electrode for radiofrequency liver ablation. Invest Radiol 2000;35:438–44.
60. Gillams AR, Lees WR. CT mapping of the distribution of saline during radiofrequency ablation with perfusion electrodes. Cardiovasc Intervent Radiol 2005;28:476–80.
61. Liu Z, Lobo SM, Humphries S, et al. Radiofrequency tumor ablation: insight into improved efficacy using computer modeling. AJR Am J Roentgenol 2005;184:1347–52.
62. Laeseke PF, Sampson LA, Winter TC 3rd, et al. Use of dextrose 5% in water instead of saline to protect against inadvertent radiofrequency injuries. AJR Am J Roentgenol 2005;184:1026–7.
63. Ahmed M, Goldberg SN. Combination radiofrequency thermal ablation and adjuvant IV liposomal doxorubicin increases tissue coagulation and intratumoural drug accumulation. Int J Hyperthermia 2004;20:781–802.
64. Horkan C, Dalal K, Coderre JA, et al. Reduced tumor growth with combined radiofrequency ablation and radiation therapy in a rat breast tumor model. Radiology 2005;235:81–8.
65. Goldberg SN, Hahn PF, Tanabe KK, et al. Percutaneous radiofrequency tissue ablation: does perfusion-mediated tissue cooling limit coagulation necrosis? J Vasc Interv Radiol 1998;9:101–11.
66. Goldberg SN, Kamel IR, Kruskal JB, et al. Radiofrequency ablation of hepatic tumors: increased tumor destruction with adjuvant liposomal doxorubicin therapy. AJR Am J Roentgenol 2002;179:93–101.

67. Head HW, Dodd GD 3rd, Bao A, et al. Combination radiofrequency ablation and intravenous radiolabeled liposomal doxorubicin: imaging and quantification of increased drug delivery to tumors. Radiology 2010;255:405–14.

68. Kang SG, Yoon CJ, Jeong SH, et al. Single-session combined therapy with chemoembolization and radiofrequency ablation in hepatocellular carcinoma less than or equal to 5 cm: a preliminary study. J Vasc Interv Radiol 2009;20: 1570–7.

69. Goldberg SN, Saldinger PF, Gazelle GS, et al. Percutaneous tumor ablation: increased coagulation necrosis with combined radiofrequency and percutaneous doxorubicin injection. Radiology 2001;220:420–7.

70. Ahmed M, Liu Z, Lukyanov AN, et al. Combination radiofrequency ablation with intratumoral liposomal doxorubicin: effect on drug accumulation and coagulation in multiple tissues and tumor types in animals. Radiology 2005;235:469–77.

71. Vaage J, Barbara E. Tissue uptake and therapeutic effects of stealth doxorubicin. In: Lasic D, Martin F, editors. Stealth liposomes. Boca Raton (FL): CRC Press, Inc; 1995.

72. Gabizon A, Shiota R, Papahadjopoulos D. Pharmacokinetics and tissue distribution of doxorubicin encapsulated in stable liposomes with long circulation times. J Natl Cancer Inst 1989;81:1484–8.

73. Ranson MR, Carmichael J, O'Byrne K, et al. Treatment of advanced breast cancer with sterically stabilized liposomal doxorubicin: results of a multicenter phase II trial. J Clin Oncol 1997;15:3185–91.

74. Gordon AN, Granai CO, Rose PG, et al. Phase II study of liposomal doxorubicin in platinum- and paclitaxel-refractory epithelial ovarian cancer. J Clin Oncol 2000; 18:3093–100.

75. Rivera E, Valero V, Arun B, et al. Phase II study of pegylated liposomal doxorubicin in combination with gemcitabine in patients with metastatic breast cancer. J Clin Oncol 2003;21:3249–54.

76. Ahmed M, Monsky WE, Girnun G, et al. Radiofrequency thermal ablation sharply increases intratumoral liposomal doxorubicin accumulation and tumor coagulation. Cancer Res 2003;63:6327–33.

77. D'Ippolito G, Ahmed M, Girnun GD, et al. Percutaneous tumor ablation: reduced tumor growth with combined radio-frequency ablation and liposomal doxorubicin in a rat breast tumor model. Radiology 2003;228:112–8.

78. Monsky WE, Goldberg SN, Lukyanov AN, et al. Radiofrequency tumor ablation increases intratumoral liposomal doxorubicin accumulation in an animal breast tumor model. Radiology 2002;224(3):823–9.

79. Poon RT, Borys N. Lyso-thermosensitive liposomal doxorubicin: a novel approach to enhance efficacy of thermal ablation of liver cancer. Expert Opin Pharmacother 2009;10:333–43.

80. Solazzo S, Ahmed M, Schor-Bardach R, et al. Liposomal doxorubicin increases radiofrequency ablation-induced tumor destruction by increasing cellular oxidative and nitrative stress and accelerating apoptotic pathways. Radiology 2010; 225(1):62–74.

81. Yang W, Ahmed M, Elian M, et al. Do liposomal apoptotic enhancers increase tumor coagulation and endpoint survival in percutaneous radiofrequency ablation of tumors in a rat tumor model? Radiology 2010;257(3):685–96.

82. Yang W, Ahmed M, Tasawwar B, et al. Radiofrequency (RF) ablation combined with adjuvant liposomal quercetin-induced heat shock protein suppression increases tumor destruction and end-point survival in a rat animal model [abstract]. Presented at the Annual Meeting of the Society of Thermal Medicine. 2010. p. 105.

83. Dromi S, Frenkel V, Luk A, et al. Pulsed-high intensity focused ultrasound and low temperature-sensitive liposomes for enhanced targeted drug delivery and anti-tumor effect. Clin Cancer Res 2007;13:2722–7.
84. Dupuy DE, DiPetrillo T, Gandhi S, et al. Radiofrequency ablation followed by conventional radiotherapy for medically inoperable stage I non-small cell lung cancer. Chest 2006;129:738–45.
85. Algan O, Fosmire H, Hynynen K, et al. External beam radiotherapy and hyper-thermia in the treatment of patients with locally advanced prostate carcinoma. Cancer 2000;89:399–403.
86. Solazzo S, Mertyna P, Peddi H, et al. RF ablation with adjuvant therapy: compar-ison of external beam radiation and liposomal doxorubicin on ablation efficacy in an animal tumor model. Int J Hyperthermia 2008;24:560–7.
87. Mayer R, Hamilton-Farrell MR, van der Kleij AJ, et al. Hyperbaric oxygen and radiotherapy. Strahlenther Onkol 2005;181:113–23.
88. Wood BJ, Kruecker J, Abi-Jaoudeh N, et al. Navigation systems for ablation. J Vasc Interv Radiol 2010;21:S257–63.
89. Krucker J, Xu S, Glossop N, et al. Electromagnetic tracking for thermal ablation and biopsy guidance: clinical evaluation of spatial accuracy. J Vasc Interv Radiol 2007;18:1141–50.
90. Klauser AS, De Zordo T, Feuchtner GM, et al. Fusion of real-time US with CT images to guide sacroiliac joint injection in vitro and in vivo. Radiology 2010; 256:547–53.
91. Khan MF, Dogan S, Maataoui A, et al. Navigation-based needle puncture of a cadaver using a hybrid tracking navigational system. Invest Radiol 2006;41: 713–20.
92. Aravalli RN, Golzarian J, Cressman EN. Animal models of cancer in interventional radiology. Eur Radiol 2009;19:1049–53.
93. Haemmerich D, Lee FT Jr. Multiple applicator approaches for radiofrequency and microwave ablation. Int J Hyperthermia 2005;21:93–106.
94. dos Santos I, Haemmerich D, Pinheiro Cda S, et al. Effect of variable heat transfer coefficient on tissue temperature next to a large vessel during radiofrequency tumor ablation. Biomed Eng Online 2008;7:21.
95. Gasselhuber A, Dreher MR, Negussie A, et al. Mathematical spatio-temporal model of drug delivery from low temperature sensitive liposomes during radiofre-quency tumour ablation. Int J Hyperthermia 2010;26:499–513.

Ablative Therapies for Colorectal Liver Metastases

Russell E. Brown, MD, Robert C.G. Martin II, MD, PhD,
Charles R. Scoggins, MD, MBA*

KEYWORDS

- Colorectal adenocarcinoma • Ablative therapies
- Liver metastases • Chemotherapy

Colorectal adenocarcinoma remains the third most common cause of cancer-related death in the United States, with an estimated 146,000 new cases and 50,000 deaths annually. Survival is stage dependent, and the presence of liver metastases is a primary determinant in patient survival. Approximately 25% of new patients present with synchronous colorectal liver metastases (CLMs), whereas up to one half develop CLMs over the course of their disease.[1–4]

The past two decades have seen significant advances in the treatment of metastatic colorectal cancer. Improvements in systemic chemotherapy have allowed for both prolonged survival and the opportunity for more patients to benefit from hepatic resection of CLM—currently, the only potentially curable treatment option. Unfortunately, because of unfavorable tumor location, disease extent, or insufficient hepatic reserve, approximately 70% of patients with CLM are not candidates for hepatic resection.[5] This has led investigators to seek alternative methods of treating those patients who are not candidates for hepatectomy. In this regard, multiple liver-directed therapies have been developed that offer an opportunity for local therapy for those patients for whom hepatic resection is not feasible.

One of the most widely accepted nonresection techniques for addressing hepatic tumors is local tumor ablation. The rationale underlying the use of local ablative therapies for metastatic colorectal cancer rests largely on the observed survival benefit after resection of CLM[6] and three theoretic concepts[7]:

1. Tumor consolidation after highly effective systemic therapy (ie, successful eradication of micrometastases with residual, stable macrometastatic burden after systemic therapy). This theory holds that elimination of this consolidated tumor may yield a survival benefit.

Division of Surgical Oncology, Department of Surgery, University of Louisville, 315 East Broadway, Suite 303, Louisville, KY 40202, USA
* Corresponding author.
E-mail address: charles.scoggins@louisville.edu

Surg Oncol Clin N Am 20 (2011) 259–271
doi:10.1016/j.soc.2010.11.005
1055-3207/11/$ – see front matter © 2011 Elsevier Inc. All rights reserved.

2. Oligometastases, that is, identification of a subgroup of patients with metastatic disease that is intermediate between completely absent and widely disseminated, which may benefit from complete ablation.[8]
3. The Norton-Simon hypothesis that effectiveness of chemotherapeutics is proportional to tumor growth rate, with the hope that tumor debulking results in a smaller-volume (and faster-growing) metastatic population of cells that are more chemosensitive.[9,10]

Nonresectional liver-directed therapies can be broadly categorized as catheter based (eg, transarterial chemoembolization, drug-eluting bead therapy, and radioembolization) or intraparenchymal ablative techniques. This review focuses on the two most widely used intraparenchymal ablative modalities for CLM by surgeons—radiofrequency ablation (RFA) and microwave ablation (MWA). A discussion of cryoablation and of emerging ablative technologies (laser interstitial thermal therapy, irreversible electroporation, and high-intensity focused ultrasound [HIFU]) is also included.

CRYOABLATION

Cryoablation was described early in the evolution of liver ablative technologies[11] and involves placement of a cryoprobe into liver metastases by open surgical, laparoscopic, or percutaneous approaches. The cryoprobe tip is then rapidly cooled using liquefied gases and, over sequential freeze-thaw cycles, forms an ice ball encompassing the CLM and a rim of normal liver. The progression of the ice ball can be easily monitored by ultrasound. Tissue destruction follows via multiple mechanisms, including membrane rupture, dehydration, protein denaturation, vascular stasis, and electrolyte disturbances.[12]

Hepatic cryoablation has some significant limitations. Heat sink effects may limit effective treatment of CLMs in close proximity to intrahepatic vascular structures, which may not allow for sufficiently low treatment temperatures. This raises the potential risk of incomplete ablation that might result in a higher risk of local recurrence. In addition, little intrinsic hemostasis is achieved by cryoablation, and hemorrhage has been reported as a result of cracking of the ice ball formation.[13,14] A potentially lethal cytokine-mediated systemic inflammatory response, termed *cryoshock*, has been described after cryoablation, with a frequency of 1%.[15,16] Perioperative mortality after cryoablation is estimated at 1.5%.[15] These complications as well as reports of inferior results compared with other ablative technologies have limited the use of cryoablation for CLMs at most centers.[17–20]

HYPERTHERMIC ABLATIVE TECHNOLOGIES

The use of hyperthermia to treat tumors dates to ancient times, with the use of cautery to treat superficial tumors.[21] Modern hyperthermic ablative technologies rely on exposure of tumors to supranormal temperatures to ablate intrahepatic tumors. In contrast to cryotherapy, where tumors are more resistant to freezing than normal cells, malignant cells are more sensitive to hyperthermic damage than normal cells.[22,23] Tumors lack the ability to dissipate heat by augmenting blood flow that is found in healthy tissues.[24]

For most tumors, exposure to temperatures above 42°C results in low-level thermal injury, with increases in injury noted with increased exposure time and temperature. At progressively higher temperatures, there is an exponential and inverse relationship between treatment temperature and the exposure time needed to achieve cell death—that is, higher treatment temperatures require less exposure time for successful ablation.[25] Temperatures above 60°C lead to reliable cell death through complex interactions, involving apoptosis, microvascular damage, ischemia-reperfusion injury, Kupffer cell activation, altered cytokine expression, alterations in the immune response, RNA and DNA destruction, dissolution of lipid bilayers, and protein denaturation.[21,26] Thermal coagulation begins at approximately 70°C, and tissue desiccation occurs at approximately 100°C.[5]

Radiofrequency Ablation of CLM

RFA achieves local hyperthermia using high-frequency alternating electric current in the radiofrequency range (100–500 kHz). Local hyperthermia results from ionic vibration and frictional heating of surrounding tissues. RFA gained popularity in the 1990s after reports by McGahan and colleagues[27] and Rossi and colleagues[28] and serves as the prototypical ablation platform for most clinicians today.

Radiofrequency current is applied through an electrode that is deployed within the tumor, using ultrasound, CT, or MRI guidance. RFA probes were initially developed as single-needle electrodes but have evolved to multiprobe and internally cooled arrays with attendant increases in treatment volumes[5] and more reliable geometric ablation zones. Several devices are marketed worldwide, and none has emerged as superior with regard to ablation size, reproducibility, or local tumor control.

Percutaneous, laparoscopic, and open surgical approaches have been successfully used for RFA treatment, each with inherent advantages and disadvantages. The choice of approach should be individualized based on tumor anatomy, extent of disease, and patient comorbidities. An open surgical approach to RFA is preferable for patients with large tumors, multiple tumors, and tumors near large blood vessels that may otherwise be inadequately ablated because of heat sink effects. Hepatic inflow occlusion (Pringle maneuver) diminishes the heat sink effect from large intrahepatic vessels and is easier with open surgery compared with laparoscopic surgery. An open approach also allows for extremely accurate intraoperative ultrasound,[29] which facilitates ablation of large tumors near blood vessels or in difficult anatomic regions of the liver. Peripherally situated tumors may be safely ablated by packing adjacent organs away from the liver, thus providing a layer of protection difficult to achieve with other approaches. Thoracic transdiaphragmatic approaches to tumors near the dome of the liver have also been described,[30] and this technique may be useful for patients in whom multiple prior surgical procedures have resulted in prohibitive perihepatic scar tissue.

Laparoscopic RFA is an option for patients with tumors for which percutaneous RFA is not feasible or safe, such as peripherally situated tumors near adjacent organs, such as the stomach or colon. Patients may benefit from the decreased incisional morbidities and faster recovery times afforded by a laparoscopic approach. Substantial surgical judgment must be exercised, however, in selecting patients for whom the laparoscopic approach is appropriate, and oncologic principles should not be compromised intraoperatively. Modern endoscopic optics and laparoscopic ultrasound probes permit excellent visualization, making this approach increasingly attractive.

Percutaneous RFA is well suited for patients with CLM who are not good candidates for more invasive procedures due to comorbid conditions. In general, percutaneous RFA requires tumor sizes and locations that can be accessed without damaging adjacent organs or vascular structures. Although CT-guided RFA is relatively easy for small tumors in the lower segments of the liver, tumors along the edge of the liver can pose exposure challenges. Artificially induced ascites or pleural effusions by injection of dextrose solution has been reported as a means of separating vulnerable nearby organs,[31–34] thus potentially expanding this indication. Cirrhotic patients and patients with limited intrahepatic recurrences after hepatectomy are examples of patients who may be best served by a percutaneous approach.

Regardless of the device or approach used, attention to RFA probe placement is critical to successful tumor ablation. Careful assessment of preablation imaging studies (CT or MRI) and thorough ultrasound examination of both the tumor and surrounding hepatic anatomy during treatment assist with successful probe placement. Ultrasonography can monitor the progression of the ablation during RFA. Gas bubbles generated by an ablation may interfere with accurate ultrasonography of tissues deep to the electrode, which can hinder repositioning of the electrode for overlapping ablation zones when treating larger tumors. Initial ablation of the deepest portions of the tumor, followed by serial redeployment as the electrode is withdrawn may mitigate this effect. Imaging-related difficulties may be more pronounced with the percutaneous approach, because transcutaneous ultrasound may not be as accurate as intraoperative ultrasonography; however, an immediate post-RFA CT can be readily performed to assist with the assessment of the ablation zone.

Complication rates associated with RFA are low, ranging from 2.4% to 27%, depending on the threshold for defining complications.[35–42] By compiling data from more than 1300 patients from 18 different studies, Scaife and Curley[43] reported an overall mortality rate of 0.5%, a major complication rate of 2%, and a minor complication rate of 6% after hepatic RFA. The risk of hepatic failure is low after RFA, even in patients with abnormal hepatic parenchyma. For this reason, RFA seems particularly attractive for cirrhotic patients. Monopolar RFA requires careful placement of grounding pads before ablation, because inadequate electrical grounding has been implicated in full-thickness skin burns.[44] Other potential complications after RFA include wound infections, intra-abdominal abscess, renal failure, hepatic abscess, biliary tract injury, pleural effusion, fever, pain, and minor hemorrhage. A postablation syndrome has also been described[45,46] and is characterized by low-grade fever, malaise, chills, myalgia, delayed pain, and nausea and vomiting. This syndrome is usually self-limited and resolves within 10 days but must be differentiated from more serious postoperative complications. Both RFA and MWA can be safely performed in patients with implanted cardiac devices but require coordination with cardiologists and perioperative device interrogation.[47]

Because there are no published randomized controlled trials comparing RFA and resection, the effectiveness of RFA in CLMs is largely based on several single-arm, retrospective or prospective studies. These studies have inherent flaws (eg, selection bias, differing endpoints, and varying definitions of eligibility for RFA or resection); however, the available data point to RFA as an effective treatment modality in improving survival in CLMs (**Box 1**). In an American Society of Clinical Oncology clinical evidence review, Wong and colleagues[48] reported wide variability in reported 5-year survival rates (14%–55%) and local recurrence rates (3.6%–60%) after RFA, which are indicative of variability in selection criteria, treatment experience/technique, and endpoints across multiple institutions.

Despite the variability in study designs, the preponderance of evidence supports the superiority of resection over RFA and a benefit of RFA over systemic chemotherapy alone. Abdalla and colleagues[49] compared 368 patients who underwent potentially curative procedures (resection only, resection with RFA, and RFA only) with 70 patients with liver-only disease who received only regional or systemic chemotherapy. This series used as a control group patients with unresectable disease confirmed at laparotomy rather than historical controls. The investigators noted significant

> **Box 1**
> **Advantages and disadvantages of RFA compared with hepatic resection**
>
> *Advantages of RFA*
>
> Lower complication rates
>
> Faster recovery
>
> Safer in patients with marginal liver reserve
>
> Ability to treat percutaneously
>
> *Disadvantages of RFA*
>
> Lack of long-term outcomes data
>
> Higher local recurrence rates
>
> Lower overall survival rates
>
> Limitations in treating large or multiple lesions

differences in both overall recurrence rates (52% [resection only] vs 64% [resection plus RFA] vs 84% [RFA only]) and 4-year survival rates (65%, 36%, and 22% for resection, resection plus RFA, and RFA only, respectively).

Abdalla and colleagues[49] reported a survival advantage for patients undergoing either resection with RFA or RFA alone compared with chemotherapy only ($P = .0017$). Also, in a series by Berber and colleagues,[50] 135 patients who were not candidates for resection treated with laparoscopic RFA, a median survival of 28.9 was longer than the historical survival of 11 to 14 months with chemotherapy alone. These data suggest that RFA, although not superior to resection, does expand the armamentarium of surgeons, allowing for treatment options beyond chemotherapy alone for patients not amenable to resection, with the potential for improved survival.

Tumor number has been shown to affect both survival and recurrence rates—patients with solitary CLM have a better outcome than those with multiple CLMs. Tumor size has been shown an important factor affecting the rate of local recurrence after RFA, with multiple groups associating CLM tumor diameter greater than or equal to 4 cm with increased rates of local recurrence.[40–42,51–53] Whether or not this is a function of unfavorable tumor biology or a limitation of current ablative technologies is a matter of ongoing debate. The relationship between increasing tumor size (or number) and increasing risk of local recurrence highlights the need for early detection and intervention for low-volume CLM.

Choice of treatment approach (open, laparoscopic, or percutaneous) may also influence local recurrence risk. Eisele and colleagues[54] and Kuvshinoff and Ota[41] reported lower rates of local recurrence for open and laparoscopic RFA versus a percutaneous approach. Improvements in hepatic exposure and the increased sensitivity of intraoperative ultrasound[55] allowed by an open or laparoscopic RFA approach likely contribute to the lower local recurrence rates after operative compared with percutaneous RFA. Additionally, open and laparoscopic approaches allow for visual inspection of the liver surface for occult lesions and of the peritoneal cavity for extrahepatic disease. The apparent superiority of operative RFA is most likely due to better visualization, better control of surrounding structures, and more sensitive inspection of the peritoneal cavity.

Microwave Ablation of CLM

MWA, like RFA, is a hyperthermic ablative modality used in the treatment of CLMs. MWA uses microwave frequencies ($\geq$900 MHz) to stimulate water molecules in target tissues, with resultant heat generation and thermal ablation.[56] Although RFA uses ionic agitation to produce heat, MWA induces rotation of water molecules with resultant rapid increases in temperature. MWA was first developed as a hemostatic adjunct to parenchymal transaction during hepatectomy.[57,58] MWA gained in popularity (largely in the Eastern hemisphere) for the treatment of hepatocellular carcinoma and later for liver metastases. Recent approval for MWA devices has led to increased use within the United States.

In clinical practice, MWA is similar to RFA in many respects, namely in selection of candidates, the device safety profile, and the approach to probe placement. Advantages of MWA include speed (median ablation times of 10 minutes), the ability to simultaneously ablate with multiple antennae, and lack of grounding pad complications.[59] Other advantages have been suggested, with regard to larger active (as opposed to conductive) heating zones and in avoiding the limitations of increased impedance around RFA probes.[60,61] **Fig. 1** shows pre- and post-MWA CT images for two CLMs treated with simultaneous application of multiple MWA antennae.

Probes for MWA include single and multiple antenna arrays as well as loop antennae for expanded ablation zones. As with RFA, MWA can be performed through percutaneous, laparoscopic (**Figs. 2** and **3**), or open surgical approaches. The reasons for choosing one approach over another parallel the rationale for RFA (discussed previously).

Although data are limited, survival and local recurrence rates after MWA seem comparable to those associated with RFA. The authors' group has reported on 50 patients with unresectable CLMs treated by MWA. At a median follow-up of 3 years, recurrences at the ablation site were noted in 6% of patients, with a median disease-free survival of 12 months and a median overall survival of 36 months.[62] As with RFA, MWA has also been employed in combination with hepatic resection for patients with CLM not amenable to one-stage resection. Tanaka and colleagues[63] reviewed 53 patients with greater than or equal to 5 bilobar CLMs who underwent either resection or resection plus MWA. At a median follow-up of 21 months, there was no significant difference between the two groups with respect to overall, disease-free, or hepatic recurrence-free survival. The 3-year overall survival was similar for patients who required combined resection/ablation and those who underwent hepatectomy alone.

Laser-Induced Thermotherapy

Laser-induced thermotherapy (LITT) is another thermal ablative technology that uses low-intensity lasers (diode or Nd:YAG) to emit photons. These photons are then

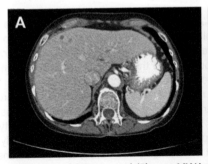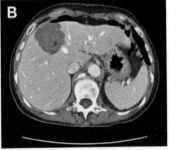

Fig. 1. CT images of (A) pre- and (B) post-MWA treatment of two CLMs.

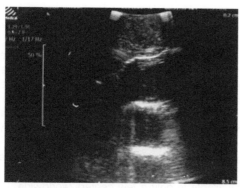

Fig. 2. Intraoperative ultrasound image of a CLM treated by laparoscopic MWA.

absorbed by natural molecular chromophores present in all human cells and converted into heat, resulting in cell death.[56,64] LITT has similar indications as RFA, namely unresectable primary and secondary liver tumors and, like RFA, can be performed by percutaneous, laparoscopic, or open surgical approaches.[65] As with other thermal ablative techniques, LITT ablation volumes can be increased by inflow occlusion, serial ablation, or placing multiple laser fibers into the target tissue, resulting in overlapping zones of ablation.[66,67]

An advantage of LITT is its compatibility with magnetic resonance guidance. Unlike RFA or MWA, LITT does not interfere with MRI. Ultrasound or CT may be used for tumor targeting and placement of the laser fibers, followed by MRI of ablation progression.[68–70] Real-time temperature monitoring is another potential advantage of LITT in conjunction with magnetic resonance guidance, because it allows clinicians to assure temperatures are high enough for successful ablation and low enough in

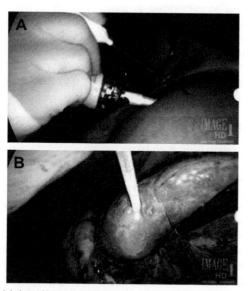

Fig. 3. Extracorporeal (A) and intracorporeal (B) intraoperative photographs of laparoscopic MWA of a CLM within segment III of the liver.

surrounding tissue to minimize collateral damage. Currently, however, the limited availability of LITT, MRI guidance, and thermal mapping has precluded widespread use of LITT.

Few large-scale studies of LITT in the treatment of CLMs have been published. Vogl and colleagues,[71] in a review of 603 patients with CLM, reported a median survival of 3.5 years and 5-year survival of 37% after diagnosis of metastases. Pech and colleagues[72] reported on 117 colorectal metastases in 66 patients treated by MRI-guided LITT. At a short median follow-up of 8.7 months, a median progression-free survival of 6.1 months and a median overall survival of 23 months were d. An analysis of the complications associated with the LITT in 899 patients with 2520 lesions (primary and metastatic) concluded that the procedure had an acceptably low morbidity, comparable to other thermal ablative modalities.[73]

Currently, LITT is available in only a few centers worldwide. Further multi-institutional studies are warranted to refine the feasibility, safety, durability, and efficacy of LITT in the treatment of CLMs.

High-Intensity Focused Ultrasound

HIFU is an emerging, noninvasive, thermal ablative technology that focuses acoustic energy within solid organs, resulting in temperature elevation and coagulative necrosis. Mechanical effects (inertial cavitation) are also observed in HIFU and contribute to cell death. HIFU transducers deliver intensities and compression/rarefaction pressures that are much higher than those seen in diagnostic ultrasound transducers.[74]

HIFU is most successful in situations with good acoustic coupling between the ultrasound probe and the tumor (eg, prostate ablation or open surgical applications in the kidney).[75] For hepatic HIFU, coupling between the skin and intervening tissues is suboptimal and has resulted in skin burns as well as rib necrosis.[76] The ablation zone after a single HIFU ablation is typically cigar shaped and measures 1 to 3 mm $\times$ 8 to 15 mm. Treatment of larger volumes requires precise painting of the target lesion[75] and can lead to difficulties in treating larger tumors in mobile organs, such as the liver. As with all thermal ablative modalities, the potential for incomplete ablation secondary to heat sink effect exists. Potential advantages of HIFU are largely related to its completely noninvasive approach. Continued refinements in techniques and technologies as well as prospective evaluations of efficacy in CLM may show it a viable future treatment option in the future.

IRREVERSIBLE ELECTROPORATION

Irreversible electroporation (IRE) is an emerging intraparenchymal ablative technology that is based on the application of short-duration (micro- to millisecond) high-voltage (1000–3000 V) pulses to target tissues, with the formation of nanoscale defects in the lipid bilayer and resultant cell necrosis.[77,78] IRE probes can be placed using open surgical, laparoscopic, or percutaneous approaches, and multiprobe arrays can be used to achieve increased ablation volumes.

IRE is unique in two respects: first, it accomplishes ablation through nonthermal means and is not hindered by heat sink effect; second, it seems that IRE preferentially ablates parenchymal tissues, with relative sparing of bile ducts and blood vessels.[79,80] These properties make IRE an attractive technology for patients with hepatic tumors in close proximity to vascular or biliary structures that would risk incomplete ablation or vascular/biliary injury with thermal ablative techniques.

Ongoing multi-institutional prospective evaluations of safety, efficacy, and durability of IRE treatments are necessary to define the patient populations most likely to benefit from this technology and to compare it with other ablative modalities.

SUMMARY

Although hepatic resection remains the gold standard therapy for CLM, many patients will continue to benefit from ablative therapies. Further refinements in techniques and technologies will continue to expand the ablative options available to patients with CLM. Continued analysis is required to delineate the biology of CLM and define the optimal role of ablation in the multidisciplinary treatment of CLM. The optimal technique for ablation of CLM should be based on patient and operator factors.

REFERENCES

1. Jemal A, Siegel R, Ward E, et al. Cancer statistics, 2009. CA Cancer J Clin 2009; 59(4):225–49.
2. Steele G Jr, Ravikumar TS. Resection of hepatic metastases from colorectal cancer. Biologic perspective. Ann Surg 1989;210(2):127–38.
3. Scheele J, Stangl R, Altendorf-Hofmann A. Hepatic metastases from colorectal carcinoma: impact of surgical resection on the natural history. Br J Surg 1990; 77(11):1241–6.
4. Lewis AM, Martin RC. The treatment of hepatic metastases in colorectal carcinoma. Am Surg 2006;72(6):466–73.
5. Parikh AA, Curley SA, Fornage BD, et al. Radiofrequency ablation of hepatic metastases. Semin Oncol 2002;29(2):168–82.
6. Tomlinson JS, Jarnagin WR, DeMatteo RP, et al. Actual 10-year survival after resection of colorectal liver metastases defines cure. J Clin Oncol 2007;25(29): 4575–80.
7. Timmerman RD, Bizekis CS, Pass HI, et al. Local surgical, ablative, and radiation treatment of metastases. CA Cancer J Clin 2009;59(3):145–70.
8. Hellman S, Weichselbaum RR. Oligometastases. J Clin Oncol 1995;13(1):8–10.
9. Norton L, Simon R. The Norton-Simon hypothesis revisited. Cancer Treat Rep 1986;70(1):163–9.
10. Simon R, Norton L. The Norton-Simon hypothesis: designing more effective and less toxic chemotherapeutic regimens. Nat Clin Pract Oncol 2006;3(8): 406–7.
11. Cooper IS, Hirose T. Application of cryogenic surgery to resection of parenchymal organs. N Engl J Med 1966;274(1):15–8.
12. Wemyss-Holden SA, Dennison AR, Berry DP, et al. Local ablation for unresectable liver tumors: is thermal best? J Hepatobiliary Pancreat Surg 2004;11(2): 97–106.
13. Onik G, Rubinsky B, Zemel R, et al. Ultrasound-guided hepatic cryosurgery in the treatment of metastatic colon carcinoma. Preliminary results. Cancer 1991;67(4): 901–7.
14. Goodie DB, Horton MD, Morris RW, et al. Anaesthetic experience with cryotherapy for treatment of hepatic malignancy. Anaesth Intensive Care 1992; 20(4):491–6.
15. Seifert JK, Morris DL. World survey on the complications of hepatic and prostate cryotherapy. World J Surg 1999;23(2):109–13 [discussion: 113–4].

16. Rodriguez-Bigas MA, Klippenstein D, Meropol NJ, et al. A pilot study of cryochemotherapy for hepatic metastases from colorectal cancer. Cryobiology 1996; 33(6):600–6.

17. Mayo SC, Pawlik TM. Thermal ablative therapies for secondary hepatic malignancies. Cancer J 2010;16(2):111–7.

18. Adam R, Akpinar E, Johann M, et al. Place of cryosurgery in the treatment of malignant liver tumors. Ann Surg 1997;225(1):39–48 [discussion: 48–50].

19. Adam R, Hagopian EJ, Linhares M, et al. A comparison of percutaneous cryosurgery and percutaneous radiofrequency for unresectable hepatic malignancies. Arch Surg 2002;137(12):1332–9 [discussion: 1340].

20. Pearson AS, Izzo F, Fleming RY, et al. Intraoperative radiofrequency ablation or cryoablation for hepatic malignancies. Am J Surg 1999;178(6):592–9.

21. Curley SA. Radiofrequency ablation of malignant liver tumors. Ann Surg Oncol 2003;10(4):338–47.

22. Steeves RA. Hyperthermia in cancer therapy: where are we today and where are we going? Bull N Y Acad Med 1992;68(2):341–50.

23. Bischof J, Christov K, Rubinsky B. A morphological study of cooling rate response in normal and neoplastic human liver tissue: cryosurgical implications. Cryobiology 1993;30(5):482–92.

24. Leveen RF. Laser hyperthermia and radiofrequency ablation of hepatic lesions. Semin Interv Radiol 1997;14:313–24.

25. Dickson JA, Calderwood SK. Temperature range and selective sensitivity of tumors to hyperthermia: a critical review. Ann N Y Acad Sci 1980;335:180–205.

26. Nikfarjam M, Muralidharan V, Christophi C. Mechanisms of focal heat destruction of liver tumors. J Surg Res 2005;127(2):208–23.

27. McGahan JP, Browning PD, Brock JM, et al. Hepatic ablation using radiofrequency electrocautery. Invest Radiol 1990;25(3):267–70.

28. Rossi S, Fornari F, Pathies C, et al. Thermal lesions induced by 480 KHz localized current field in guinea pig and pig liver. Tumori 1990;76(1):54–7.

29. Scaife CL, Ng CS, Ellis LM, et al. Accuracy of preoperative imaging of hepatic tumors with helical computed tomography. Ann Surg Oncol 2006; 13(4):542–6.

30. Mullen JT, Walsh GL, Abdalla EK, et al. Transdiaphragmatic radiofrequency ablation of liver tumors. J Am Coll Surg 2004;199(5):826–9.

31. Raman SS, Lu DS, Vodopich DJ, et al. Minimizing diaphragmatic injury during radio-frequency ablation: efficacy of subphrenic peritoneal saline injection in a porcine model. Radiology 2002;222(3):819–23.

32. Laeseke PF, Sampson LA, Winter TC 3rd, et al. Use of dextrose 5% in water instead of saline to protect against inadvertent radiofrequency injuries. AJR Am J Roentgenol 2005;184(3):1026–7.

33. Laeseke PF, Sampson LA, Brace CL, et al. Unintended thermal injuries from radiofrequency ablation: protection with 5% dextrose in water. AJR Am J Roentgenol 2006;186(Suppl 5):S249–54.

34. Head HW, Dodd GD 3rd, Dalrymple NC, et al. Percutaneous radiofrequency ablation of hepatic tumors against the diaphragm: frequency of diaphragmatic injury. Radiology 2007;243(3):877–84.

35. Curley SA, Izzo F, Delrio P, et al. Radiofrequency ablation of unresectable primary and metastatic hepatic malignancies: results in 123 patients. Ann Surg 1999; 230(1):1–8.

36. Bowles BJ, Machi J, Limm WM, et al. Safety and efficacy of radiofrequency thermal ablation in advanced liver tumors. Arch Surg 2001;136(8):864–9.

37. Wong SL, Edwards MJ, Chao C, et al. Radiofrequency ablation for unresectable hepatic tumors. Am J Surg 2001;182(6):552–7.
38. Iannitti DA, Dupuy DE, Mayo-Smith WW, et al. Hepatic radiofrequency ablation. Arch Surg 2002;137(4):422–6 [discussion: 427].
39. Jiang HC, Liu LX, Piao DX, et al. Clinical short-term results of radiofrequency ablation in liver cancers. World J Gastroenterol 2002;8(4):624–30.
40. Kosari K, Gomes M, Hunter D, et al. Local, intrahepatic, and systemic recurrence patterns after radiofrequency ablation of hepatic malignancies. J Gastrointest Surg 2002;6(2):255–63.
41. Kuvshinoff BW, Ota DM. Radiofrequency ablation of liver tumors: influence of technique and tumor size. Surgery 2002;132(4):605–11 [discussion: 611–2].
42. Bleicher RJ, Allegra DP, Nora DT, et al. Radiofrequency ablation in 447 complex unresectable liver tumors: lessons learned. Ann Surg Oncol 2003;10(1):52–8.
43. Scaife CL, Curley SA. Complication, local recurrence, and survival rates after radiofrequency ablation for hepatic malignancies. Surg Oncol Clin N Am 2003;12(1):243–55.
44. Goldberg SN. Radiofrequency tumor ablation: principles and techniques. Eur J Ultrasound 2001;13(2):129–47.
45. Dodd GD 3rd, Napier D, Schoolfield JD, et al. Percutaneous radiofrequency ablation of hepatic tumors: postablation syndrome. AJR Am J Roentgenol 2005;185(1):51–7.
46. Wah TM, Arellano RS, Gervais DA, et al. Image-guided percutaneous radiofrequency ablation and incidence of post-radiofrequency ablation syndrome: prospective survey. Radiology 2005;237(3):1097–102.
47. Skonieczki BD, Wells C, Wasser EJ, et al. Radiofrequency and microwave tumor ablation in patients with implanted cardiac devices: is it safe? Eur J Radiol 2010. [Epub ahead of print].
48. Wong SL, Mangu PB, Choti MA, et al. American Society of Clinical Oncology 2009 clinical evidence review on radiofrequency ablation of hepatic metastases from colorectal cancer. J Clin Oncol 2010;28(3):493–508.
49. Abdalla EK, Vauthey JN, Ellis LM, et al. Recurrence and outcomes following hepatic resection, radiofrequency ablation, and combined resection/ablation for colorectal liver metastases. Ann Surg 2004;239(6):818–25 [discussion: 825–7].
50. Berber E, Pelley R, Siperstein AE. Predictors of survival after radiofrequency thermal ablation of colorectal cancer metastases to the liver: a prospective study. J Clin Oncol 2005;23(7):1358–64.
51. Wood TF, Rose DM, Chung M, et al. Radiofrequency ablation of 231 unresectable hepatic tumors: indications, limitations, and complications. Ann Surg Oncol 2000;7(8):593–600.
52. Machi J, Uchida S, Sumida K, et al. Ultrasound-guided radiofrequency thermal ablation of liver tumors: percutaneous, laparoscopic, and open surgical approaches. J Gastrointest Surg 2001;5(5):477–89.
53. Chan RP, Asch M, Kachura J, et al. Radiofrequency ablation of malignant hepatic neoplasms. Can Assoc Radiol J 2002;53(5):272–8.
54. Eisele RM, Neumann U, Neuhaus P, et al. Open surgical is superior to percutaneous access for radiofrequency ablation of hepatic metastases. World J Surg 2009;33(4):804–11.
55. van Vledder MG, Pawlik TM, Munireddy S, et al. Factors determining the sensitivity of intraoperative ultrasonography in detecting colorectal liver metastases in the modern era. Ann Surg Oncol 2010;17(10):2756–63.

56. Izzo F. Other thermal ablation techniques: microwave and interstitial laser ablation of liver tumors. Ann Surg Oncol 2003;10(5):491–7.
57. Tabuse K, Katsumi M. Application of a microwave tissue coagulator to hepatic surgery the hemostatic effects on spontaneous rupture of hepatoma and tumor necrosis. Nippon Geka Hokan 1981;50(4):571–9.
58. Tabuse K, Katsumi M, Kobayashi Y, et al. Microwave surgery: hepatectomy using a microwave tissue coagulator. World J Surg 1985;9(1):136–43.
59. Martin RC, Scoggins CR, McMasters KM. Microwave hepatic ablation: initial experience of safety and efficacy. J Surg Oncol 2007;96(6):481–6.
60. Skinner MG, Iizuka MN, Kolios MC, et al. A theoretical comparison of energy sources–microwave, ultrasound and laser–for interstitial thermal therapy. Phys Med Biol 1998;43(12):3535–47.
61. Wright AS, Lee FT Jr, Mahvi DM. Hepatic microwave ablation with multiple antennae results in synergistically larger zones of coagulation necrosis. Ann Surg Oncol 2003;10(3):275–83.
62. Martin RC, Scoggins CR, McMasters KM. Safety and efficacy of microwave ablation of hepatic tumors: a prospective review of a 5-year experience. Ann Surg Oncol 2010;17(1):171–8.
63. Tanaka K, Shimada H, Nagano Y, et al. Outcome after hepatic resection versus combined resection and microwave ablation for multiple bilobar colorectal metastases to the liver. Surgery 2006;139(2):263–73.
64. Muralidharan V, Christophi C. Interstitial laser thermotherapy in the treatment of colorectal liver metastases. J Surg Oncol 2001;76(1):73–81.
65. Germer CT, Albrecht D, Roggan A, et al. Technology for in situ ablation by laparoscopic and image-guided interstitial laser hyperthermia. Semin Laparosc Surg 1998;5(3):195–203.
66. Sturesson C, Liu DL, Stenram U, et al. Hepatic inflow occlusion increases the efficacy of interstitial laser-induced thermotherapy in rat. J Surg Res 1997;71(1):67–72.
67. Heisterkamp J, van Hillegersberg R, Ijzermans JN. Interstitial laser coagulation for hepatic tumours. Br J Surg 1999;86(3):293–304.
68. Vogl TJ, Muller PK, Hammerstingl R, et al. Malignant liver tumors treated with MR imaging-guided laser-induced thermotherapy: technique and prospective results. Radiology 1995;196(1):257–65.
69. Dick EA, Joarder R, de Jode M, et al. MR-guided laser thermal ablation of primary and secondary liver tumours. Clin Radiol 2003;58(2):112–20.
70. Dick EA, Wragg P, Joarder R, et al. Feasibility of abdomino-pelvic T1-weighted real-time thermal mapping of laser ablation. J Magn Reson Imaging 2003;17(2):197–205.
71. Vogl TJ, Straub R, Eichler K, et al. Colorectal carcinoma metastases in liver: laser-induced interstitial thermotherapy—local tumor control rate and survival data. Radiology 2004;230(2):450–8.
72. Pech M, Wieners G, Freund T, et al. MR-guided interstitial laser thermotherapy of colorectal liver metastases: efficiency, safety and patient survival. Eur J Med Res 2007;12(4):161–8.
73. Vogl TJ, Straub R, Eichler K, et al. Malignant liver tumors treated with MR imaging-guided laser-induced thermotherapy: experience with complications in 899 patients (2,520 lesions). Radiology 2002;225(2):367–77.
74. Padma S, Martinie JB, Iannitti DA. Liver tumor ablation: percutaneous and open approaches. J Surg Oncol 2009;100(8):619–34.
75. Kennedy JE. High-intensity focused ultrasound in the treatment of solid tumours. Nat Rev Cancer 2005;5(4):321–7.

76. Jung SE, Cho SH, Jang JH, et al. High-intensity focused ultrasound ablation in hepatic and pancreatic cancer: complications. Abdom Imaging 2010. [Epub ahead of print].
77. Davalos RV, Mir IL, Rubinsky B. Tissue ablation with irreversible electroporation. Ann Biomed Eng 2005;33(2):223–31.
78. Miller L, Leor J, Rubinsky B. Cancer cells ablation with irreversible electroporation. Technol Cancer Res Treat 2005;4(6):699–705.
79. Edd JF, Horowitz L, Davalos RV, et al. In vivo results of a new focal tissue ablation technique: irreversible electroporation. IEEE Trans Biomed Eng 2006;53(7): 1409–15.
80. Rubinsky B, Onik G, Mikus P. Irreversible electroporation: a new ablation modality–clinical implications. Technol Cancer Res Treat 2007;6(1):37–48.

Radiofrequency Ablation of Neuroendocrine Hepatic Metastasis

T. Clark Gamblin, MD, MS*, Kathleen Christians, MD,
Sam G. Pappas, MD

KEYWORDS

- Liver cancer • Neuroendocrine cancer
- Radiofrequency ablation

Metastasis of neuroendocrine tumors varies according to the primary diagnosis and is reported to occur as frequently in 75% of glucagonomas to as rare as 5% to 10% of carcinoid tumors.[1] Tumors generally advance in an indolent predictable pattern that allows multiple therapeutic options. Although the reported incidence of neuroendocrine tumors in the United States is only 1 to 2 per 100,000 people, more than half the patients with clinically apparent tumor have or will develop liver metastases.[2] Surgery remains the primary therapy through either cytoreductive debulking or curative resection. The introduction of radiofrequency ablation (RFA) has allowed physicians to surgically address a larger population of patients with a curative intent ablation alone, or in combination with resection. Reports to date regarding RFA management are largely single-institution retrospective series.[3–5] This article provides a brief summary of the types of neuroendocrine tumors and therapies, with focus on RFA of neuroendocrine hepatic metastases.

GASTROINTESTINAL NEUROENDOCRINE NEOPLASMS

The gastrointestinal tract is the most common site for carcinoid tumors to occur, with the most common specific sites being the appendix, small intestine, and rectum.[6] Appendiceal tumors are typically small with most less than 1 cm and are primarily managed by routine appendectomy. Rectal carcinoids are also typically less aggressive and often managed by local excision alone.[7]

The authors have nothing to disclose regarding this manuscript.
Medical College of Wisconsin, Division of Surgical Oncology, 9200 West Wisconsin Avenue, Milwaukee, WI 53226–3596, USA
* Corresponding author.
E-mail address: tcgamblin@mcw.edu

Surg Oncol Clin N Am 20 (2011) 273–279
doi:10.1016/j.soc.2010.11.002
1055-3207/11/$ – see front matter © 2011 Elsevier Inc. All rights reserved.

The most common and clinically threatening site of origin for carcinoid is the small intestine. These tumors are the most frequent to involve the liver at presentation, and liver metastasis eventually develop in up to 85% of cases.[8]

In advanced cases, carcinoid syndrome may occur characterized by flushing, diarrhea, asthma, bronchospasm, or in very advanced cases, carcinoid heart disease. This unique symptomatic expression typically occurs in 35% to 50% of patients with hepatic disease.[9] Most patients have increased serotonin production and the levels of urinary 5-hydroxyindoleacetic acid are directly related to the severity of symptoms. Typically these cancers are very slow growing and duration of disease from diagnosis to eventual death is more than 9 years. The tumor has accurately been described as "cancer in slow motion." In those with unresectable disease, 5-year median survival is reported to approach 30%.[7]

ISLET CELL NEOPLASMS

Pancreatic islet cell tumors are functional in about 50% of cases and typically produce more than 1 hormone. Neoplasms are named for the dominant hormone produced, such as insulinoma, gastrinoma, glucagonoma, VIPoma, and somatostatinoma. Considerable morbidity and mortality may occur as a result of the production of the dominant hormone. The severity of the syndrome is proportional to the overall tumor burden.[10]

These tumors also frequently metastasize to the liver with incidence varying by type. Metastases most commonly occur in gastrinomas and least frequently in insulinomas.[11] Despite the potential for severe symptoms, the clinical course of patients even in the presence of distant metastases, can be quite indolent with 5-year survival approaching 30%.[12]

TREATMENT OF NEUROENDOCRINE HEPATIC METASTASES

Surgical intervention is considered the first choice for management, however many patients present with a disease burden or hepatic parenchymal location that prevents curative surgery or cytoreductive surgery.[11] Somatostatin analogues, hepatic artery embolization, and systemic chemotherapy are also used depending on the location of the primary, systemic symptoms, and feasibility of surgery.

SURGICAL RESECTION

When technically possible, resection of the primary and the liver metastases affords the greatest survival advantage. Hepatic tumors are often well circumscribed rather than infiltrative and thus liver resection may be a feasible option with acceptable margins.

Patients with metastatic disease are assessed for resection with high-quality magnetic resonance imaging (MRI) or computed tomography (CT). Resection of the primary and 90% of the metastatic disease is the proposed goal for surgical intervention.[13] This strategy of aggressive resection has produced 5-year survival rates of approximately 60%. One retrospective study even reported a median survival of 7 years, and because of slow growth of the tumor, 35% were alive at 10 years.[14]

Most patients present with advanced bilobar disease and approximately 10% are considered for surgical resection alone. In addition to advanced bilobar disease, approximately 45% of patients possess concurrent extrahepatic disease. Surgical intervention is complex often involving concurrent primary tumor resection. Mortality ranges up to 6%, with complications occurring in 5% to 30% of cases.[15]

Survival of those treated with cytoreductive intent is similar to those resected with curative intent. Survival is also comparable in metastatic carcinoid and islet cell tumors and hormonally active metastatic disease does not portend a worse outcome.

Surgical resection has been shown to provide superior 5-year survival in selected patients when compared with medical or hepatic artery embolization therapy. Blumgart and colleagues[15] reported 76% 5-year survival in a surgical group compared with 53% in an embolization group, but no survivors with medical management alone. Symptom control may be gained with the surgical resection and is reported to improve in 96% to 100% of cases with a median time to symptom recurrence of 45 months. Long-term recurrence after resection is very high and some have predicted disease will recur in all patients by 7.5 years.

Liver transplantation is only considered in highly selected patients with a previously controlled primary tumor and no extrahepatic disease. However, even in carefully selected patients, recurrence is high. In a review of 103 patients, overall 5-year survival was 47% and recurrence-free survival was only 24%.[16]

HEPATIC ARTERY EMBOLIZATION

In patients who are deemed unresectable, hepatic artery embolization may offer an effective palliative approach. Because these hypervascular tumors are primarily fed by the hepatic artery rather than the portal vein, the hepatic artery provides unique access to the tumor. This regional approach does not prevent subsequent surgery or concurrent systemic therapy and response rates of 50% to 96% have been reported. Duration of the response has been the greatest challenge to this treatment option with reports ranging from 4 to 18 months.[17,18]

MEDICAL THERAPY

Somatostatin analogues are the first-line systemic agent used in the management of functioning neuroendocrine tumors. These analogues bind to the somatostatin receptors that are present on most neuroendocrine tumor cells.[19] These agents have been shown to effectively control symptoms and improve quality of life for most patients.[20] Recent evidence from the randomized PROVID study shows that analogues have affected progression-free survival, but overall survival was not significantly changed.[21] Cytotoxic agents are less effective primarily because neuroendocrine tumors are well-differentiated and have a low proliferative index.[22]

RADIOFREQUENCY ABLATION

RFA is the primary modality used currently for ablation for neuroendocrine metastases to the liver.[23,24] The introduction of RFA has allowed for intraoperative destruction of lesions and/or recurrences. Technologic advances such as the internally cooled ablation tips have made delivery more efficient and effective.[25] Laparoscopic and percutaneous approaches have also minimized morbidity associated with treatment. Ultrasound guidance is the standard of care to identify lesions of interest and confirm proper ablation probe placement. Based on the surgical experience of debulking resulting in improved survival and symptoms, ablations that destroy more than 90% of the tumor burden are now considered. The greatest success in ablation is noted in smaller lesions and thus appropriate selection of cases for RFA is vital. Although other forms of ablation exist such as ethanol injection or more recently, microwave ablation, our discussion in this article is focused on RFA.

There are no prospective trials showing survival advantage for RFA management of neuroendocrine cancer, however several retrospective analyses have indicated a seemingly clear benefit of RFA for symptom relief and survival for various types of cancer.[4,14]

Berber and colleagues[26] have published large series of hepatic neuroendocrine tumors undergoing RFA. They have reported 234 ablations in 34 patients and achieved symptom relief in 95% of cases with a median duration of 10 months. Decreased levels of at least 1 hormone marker were noted in 65% of patients. New liver metastases developed in 28% at a mean follow-up of 1.6 years. Local recurrence at the ablation site was noted to occur in only 3% of treated metastasis sites.

The symptom response to RFA has been documented in other series as well and may allow patients to discontinue the use of octreotide therapy to control carcinoid symptoms. RFA has also been reported in patients unresponsive to hepatic artery embolization allowing octreotide to be decreased or discontinued.[5]

Hellman and colleagues[27] reported 21 patients undergoing 43 ablations with an intraoperative or percutaneous approach. Mean size of tumor was 2 cm and 15 patients were treated with curative intent. At 2-year follow-up, 95% were without evidence of disease. Although there is little chance of cure, the treatment of liver metastasis remains important both for control of symptoms and slow progression.[28]

Hepatic resection remains the standard of care for patients, however RFA is an important therapeutic option (**Box 1**). Superficial tumors are not ideal for RFA, as they can be enucleated easily with minimal loss of hepatic function. The number of lesions or their location are the primary reasons few patients are resection candidates. Complementary ablation extends the group of patients for operative management as it can be used alone, or combined with liver resection. RFA allows for more aggressive management of small foci of disease deep within the liver in turn voiding major resection. This approach minimizes the surrounding parenchymal loss protecting the necessary hepatic reserve (**Fig. 1**).

Patients with extensive comorbidities or extensive tumor burden may not be surgical candidates. RFA may be performed percutaneously and thus offers an important option to potentially prolong survival. Patients who have undergone prior liver surgery should be considered for percutaneous ablation. This approach allows for subsequent treatment sessions when the tumor eventually recurs.

Operator experience is incredibly important when interpreting RFA results. Poon and colleagues[29] have reported on the learning curve of RFA describing the first 100 patients receiving RFA at their institution. They demonstrated that the second half of the series had a shorter procedure time, shorter hospital stay, fewer complications, and a 100% complete ablation rate compared with 84% in the earlier half of the

---

Box 1
Considerations for RFA of neuroendocrine hepatic metastases

1. Adjunct with liver resection

2. Treatment of patients who are not resection candidates

3. Palliation of carcinoid syndrome symptoms

4. Management of recurrent disease after resection or prior ablation

5. Ablation of deep small lesions to minimize the normal parenchyma resected

6. Most successful ablation is in lesions ≤ 3 cm

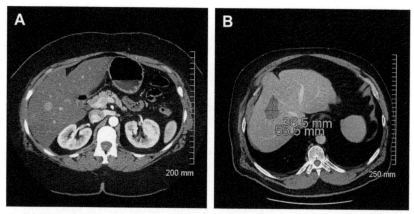

Fig. 1. (*A*) Patient with a 1.2-cm metastatic carcinoid lesion deep in the right hepatic lobe. Characteristic hypervascular component is seen on the triphasic CT scan. Relatively small left hepatic lobe is noted and ultrasound-guided ablation is performed. (*B*) CT scan 3 months after ablation shows no recurrence of disease and patient will be surveyed with subsequent imaging every 3 months for the first 2 years.

series. This learning curve is important when comparing investigators' experiences and results with RFA.

Mazzaglia and colleagues[28] have demonstrated that on multivariate analysis, the size of the dominant lesion is a strong predictor of mortality and patients with dominant tumors larger than 3 cm had a worse prognosis. In their series, women also had a better prognosis than men. The finding may be related to the biology of the disease and is conceptually similar to thyroid cancer where women have a better prognosis. Patient and tumor characteristics that did not affect survival included age, tumor type, number of lesions, number of RFA sessions, tumor markers, and presence of symptoms.

Siperstein and Berber[3] recently reported their 10-year experience using RFA for neuroendocrine hepatic metastases. Sixty-three patients underwent a total of 452 laparoscopic ablations. No resections were performed. Twenty-two percent underwent repeat ablation for progression of disease. Median survival was 11 years from diagnosis of the primary, 5.5 years after diagnosis of the hepatic metastases, and 3.9 years after the first RFA. Five-year survival was 48% and is comparable to the 61% reported by Sarmiento and colleagues[14] after aggressive surgical resection.

SUMMARY

Neuroendocrine tumors are indolent tumors of the gastrointestinal tract but are relentless in their growth. Surgical resection is the gold standard for management. RFA allows inclusion of additional patients for surgical management, resulting in improved symptom control, quality of life, and prolonged overall survival. Studies to date have shown excellent local tumor control and low morbidity with RFA. Preoperative CT and/or MRI coupled with intraoperative ultrasonography help guide localization for RFA. On the horizon are new image-guidance systems that allow three-dimensional images in the operating room. This technology will allow confirmation of probe placement in a uniform manner and may enhance outcomes.

REFERENCES

1. Siperstein AE, Berber E. Cryoablation, percutaneous alcohol injection, and radio-frequency ablation for treatment of neuroendocrine liver metastases. World J Surg 2001;25:693–6.
2. Maithel SK, Fong Y. Hepatic ablation of neuroendocrine tumor metastases. J Surg Oncol 2009;100(8):635–8.
3. Berber E, Siperstein A. Local recurrence after laparoscopic radiofrequency abla-tion of liver tumors: an analysis of 1032 tumors. Ann Surg Oncol 2008;15(10): 2757–64.
4. Atwell TD, Charboneau JW, Que FG, et al. Treatment of neuroendocrine cancer metastatic to the liver: the role of ablative techniques. Cardiovasc Intervent Radiol 2005;28:409–21.
5. Henn AR, Levine EA, McNulty W, et al. Percutaneous radiofrequency ablation of hepatic metastases for symptomatic relief of neuroendocrine syndromes. Am J Roentgenol 2003;181:1005–10.
6. Modlin IM, Sandor A. An analysis of 8305 cases of carcinoid tumors. Cancer 1997;79:813–29.
7. Moertel CG. Karnofsky memorial lecture: an odyssey in the land of small tumors. J Clin Oncol 1987;5:1502–22.
8. Ihse I, Persson B, Tibblin S. Neuroendocrine metastases of the liver. World J Surg 1995;19:76–82.
9. Shebani KO, Souba WW, Finkelstein DN, et al. Prognosis and survival in patients with gastrointestinal tract carcinoid tumors. Ann Surg 1999;229:815–22.
10. Capella C, Heitz PU, Hofler H, et al. Revised classification of neuroendocrine tumours of the lung, pancreas and gut. Virchows Arch 1995;425:547–60.
11. Carty SE, Jensen RT, Norton JA. Prospective study of aggressive resection of metastatic pancreatic endocrine tumors. Surgery 1992;112:1024–31.
12. Chen H, Hardacre JM, Uzar A, et al. Isolated liver metastases from neuroendo-crine tumors: does resection prolong survival? J Am Coll Surg 1998;187:88–92.
13. Que FG, Nagorney DM, Batts KP, et al. Hepatic resection for metastatic neuroen-docrine carcinomas. Am J Surg 1995;169:36–42.
14. Sarmiento JM, Heywood G, Rubin J, et al. Surgical treatment of neuroendocrine metastases to the liver: a plea for resection to increase survival. J Am Coll Surg 2003;197:29–37.
15. Chamberlain RS, Canes D, Brown KT, et al. Hepatic neuroendocrine metastases: does intervention alter outcomes? J Am Coll Surg 2000;190:432–45.
16. Knechtle SJ, Kalayoglu M, D'Alessandro AM, et al. Proceed with caution: liver transplantation for metastatic neuroendocrine tumors. Ann Surg 1997;225:345–6.
17. Proye C. Natural history of liver metastasis of gastrenteropancreatic tract carci-noid tumors: place for chemoembolization. World J Surg 2001;25:685–8.
18. Brown KT, Koh BY, Brody LA, et al. Particle embolization of hepatic neuroendo-crine metastases for control of pain and hormonal symptoms. J Vasc Interv Radiol 1999;10:397–403.
19. Janson ET, Westlin JE, Eriksson B, et al. In[111] octreotide scintigraphy in patients with carcinoid tumours: the predictive value of somatostatin analogue treatment. Eur J Endocrinol 1994;131:577–81.
20. Oberg K. Chemotherapy and biotherapy in the treatment of neuroendocrine tumours. Ann Oncol 2001;12(Suppl 2):S111–4.
21. Rinke A, Muller HH, Schade-Brittinger C, et al. Placebo-controlled, double blind, prospective, randomized study on the effect of octreotide in the control of tumor

growth in patients with metastatic neuroendocrine midgut tumors: a report from the PROMID study group. J Clin Oncol 2009;27(28):4656–63.

22. Bajetta E, Ferrari L, Procopio G, et al. Efficacy of a chemotherapy combination for the treatment of metastatic neuroendocrine tumours. Ann Oncol 2002;13:614–21.
23. Bowles BJ, Machi J, Limm WM, et al. Safety and efficacy of radiofrequency thermal ablation in advanced liver tumors. Arch Surg 2001;136:864–9.
24. Curley SA, Izzo F, Delrio P, et al. Radiofrequency ablation of unresectable primary and metastatic hepatic malignancies: results in 123 patients. Ann Surg 1999;230: 1–8.
25. Gillams AR. Liver ablation therapy. Br J Radiol 2004;77:713–23.
26. Berber E, Fleshner N, Siperstein AE. Laparoscopic radiofrequency ablation of neuroendocrine liver metastases. World J Surg 2002;26:985–90.
27. Hellman P, Ladjevardi S, Skogseid B, et al. Radiofrequency tissue ablation using cooled tip for liver metastases of endocrine tumors. World J Surg 2002;26: 1052–6.
28. Mazzaglia PJ, Berber E, Siperstein AE. Radiofrequency thermal ablation of meta-static neuroendocrine tumors in the liver. Curr Treat Options Oncol 2007;8: 322–30.
29. Poon RT, Ng KK, Lam CM, et al. Learning curve for radiofrequency ablation of liver tumors: prospective analysis of initial 100 patients in a tertiary institution. Ann Surg 2004;239:441–9.

Radiofrequency Ablation of Hepatocellular Carcinoma

Tito Livraghi, MD*

KEYWORDS

- Hepatocellular carcinoma • Radiofrequency ablation
- Percutaneous ablation procedure

Advances in diagnostic imaging and fine-needle biopsy technique have permitted the development of percutaneous ablation therapies (PATs). These therapies are performed using a direct image-guided approach through the skin and organ parenchyma. PATs may be based on the use of means capable of destroying the tissue chemically, such as ethyl alcohol (PEI) or acetic acid (PAI), or physically, such as laser, radiofrequency (RF), or microwave (MW). These techniques permit the destruction of tumors without necessitating their removal and, in some cases, can be used in place of more invasive and expensive surgical procedures.

PEI, the first PAT to be proposed, was independently conceived at the University of Chiba in Japan and at the Vimercate Hospital (Milan) in Italy. The first study in an international journal appeared in 1986.[1] From its rationale and the results obtained, the other techniques were subsequently designed.[2–5] Whereas for some years only patients with up to 3 small (3 cm in size) or single (<5 cm in size) lesions were treated, and this still applies at many centers, with the introduction of single-session procedures under general anesthesia,[6] even patients with lesions greater in number or larger in size are now being treated.

RF ablation (RFA) is currently considered the gold standard among PATs because of its recent results. In the clinical field, RFA is used for the treatment of a variety of neoplasms, principally metastatic hepatic deposits, hepatocellular carcinoma (HCC) in cirrhosis, renal cell carcinoma, lung tumors, and osteoid osteoma.

This article considers RFA of HCC in patients with cirrhosis. In this disease, this minimally invasive therapy has the potential to dramatically alter patient outcome, because other existing therapies either are associated with significant morbidity, or

The author has nothing to disclose.
Interventional Radiology Department, Istituto Clinico Humanitas, Rozzano (Milano), Italy
* Via Manzoni 56, 20089 Rozzano (Milano), Italy.
E-mail address: lalivra@tin.it

Surg Oncol Clin N Am 20 (2011) 281–299
doi:10.1016/j.soc.2010.11.010
1055-3207/11/$ – see front matter © 2011 Published by Elsevier Inc.

have limited efficacy. In these patients, liver dysfunction and associated coagulopathy often combine to make surgical resection an unacceptably risky procedure.

PRINCIPLES AND TECHNIQUES

The treatment of thermoablation with RF exploits the conversion of the energy of an electromagnetic wave into heat. A generator is used that converts normal energy supplied by an electric alternating current of 90 Hz into the RF band of 500 KHz. The current is linked to an active electrode in the form of a needle, which is inserted into the tumor so that the body becomes part of the electric circuit, and is dispersed with a passive electrode in the form of a plate, which is applied to the skin of the patient. In this way, a resistive type of heating is produced, particularly around the exposed point of the needle electrode, caused by ionic agitation of the tissue electrolytes that follow the change in direction of the alternating current. Heat is generated by means of impedance (resistance) that the surrounding tissue opposes to the flow of current, so that heat is not generated at the tip of the electrode but within the tissue. The heat is produced by the difference between the heat generated around the extremity of the electrode and dispersed heat, the entity of which depends on the conductivity of the tissue and dissipation by convection caused by blood circulation (the so-called sink effect). In the presence of a physical and electrical homogeneity, the heat generated around the noninsulated extremity of the electrode is regulated by the distance from the tip, by the intensity of the current, and by the duration of the application. One potential limitation of conventional monopolar RF techniques is that the diameter of tissue coagulated is limited by heat dispersion to a maximum of approximately 1.6 cm. Increasing tip temperatures to greater than 100°C does not result in greater volumes of coagulation necrosis, because of tissue vaporization and charring. This situation leads to increased local tissue impedance and thereby limits RF deposition, heat diffusion, and coagulation necrosis. To overcome these limitations, several strategies have been proposed. These strategies include the use of bipolar electrodes, multiprobe arrays, saline injection during treatment, and cooled-tip electrodes.

RFA EQUIPMENT

Several generators are commercially available, some of which have incorporated circuitry that enables measurements of generator output (wattage and milliamperage), tissue impedance, and electrode tip temperature. The most widely used instruments are made by 3 companies: RadioTherapeutics Corporation (Sunnyvale, CA, USA), acquired by Boston Scientific; RITA Medical Systems (Mountain View, CA, USA), acquired by AngioDynamics; and Radionics (Burlington, MA, USA), acquired by Covidien, a division of Tyco Healthcare Group. Each of the devices uses a different needle design, wattage, and algorithms.[3,7–9] The first uses different LeVeen electrodes capable of obtaining ablations 2 to 5 cm in size with an expandable umbrella-shaped array design, 1.9 mm in diameter. The electrodes are available with array diameter ranging from 2.0 to 5.0 cm. The RF 2000 and the RF 3000 generators produce maximum powers of 100 and 200 W, respectively. The second produced different models with time. The Starburst ablation device has a unique patented umbrella-shaped array design with a live trocar tip, 9 electrodes, and produces real-time temperature feedback from 5 independent thermocouples within the array. The 1500X RF generator has a maximal 250-W power output. The generator is started at 25 W and slowly increased over a few minutes. Once the temperature is around 100°C, the hooks are fully deployed. The main difference between the 2 systems is that LeVeen model uses tissue impedance as feedback monitoring, whereas the RITA model relies on temperature. The third uses a single cold perfusion electrode with a diameter of 1.2 mm and the tip exposed for 2 to 3 cm. The power RF generator has a maximal 20-W power output and can display temperature as well as tissue impedance. By avoiding early increments of impedance linked to carbonization, these electrodes permit application of a greater power with respect to conventional electrodes. To obtain cooling, a physiologic solution brought to 2 to 5°C is circulated within 2 coaxial lumens situated in the electrode. The technique determines a reproducible area of necrosis of 2 to 4 cm in diameter. An electrode with a cluster of 3 cooled tips in a triangular pattern, permitting a higher current deposition, determines more than 4.5 cm of coagulation necrosis.[10]

Two prospective trials compared the effectiveness of RFA performed by using different models for the treatment of HCC until 3.0 cm in size. Shibata and colleagues[11] performed a comparison of Cool-tip single electrode and LeVeen electrode with 10 expandable hooks. There was no significant difference in local effectiveness, major complications, local tumor progression, and overall survival (OS). Lin and colleagues[12] performed a comparison of the RF 2000 with LeVeen electrode, RF 3000 with LeVeen electrode, RITA with StarBurst electrode, and Cool-tip single electrode for the ablation of HCC. Similarly, there was no significant difference in the rate of volume necrosis obtained, in the rate of local tumor progression, in overall and disease-free survival at 2 years, between the groups.

Other instruments are made by Invatec (Concesio, Italy), recently acquired by Medtronic Inc, producing an electrode containing 1 or 3 spiral arrays that when deployed extend 2.0 cm beyond the tip, and Celon AG (Berlin, Germany), a member of the Olympus Medical System Group, producing a bipolar or multipolar electrode that avoids the use of the passive pad placed on the patient's thigh.

PROCEDURE

RFA is generally performed percutaneously under ultrasound (US) guidance, because this real-time control allows faster execution, precise centering of the electrode on the target, continuous monitoring of distribution of vapor bubbles, and determination of the appropriate amount of energy to give each time. A hyperechoic focus, which represents microbubbles of gas that form in the heated tissue, increases in size during the procedure, starting from the distal part of the uninsulated tip and then occupying the target. This region can be variable in size and irregular in shape and contour, and grossly reproduces the area of necrosis obtained. This hyperechogenicity obscures the tumor for 10 to 15 minutes after treatment, and sometimes makes it difficult to reposition the electrode for further insertions in brief time. Second-generation US contrast media injected after treatment are useful to decide on persistence of viable tissue. In some centers, principally in the United States, the procedure is performed under computed tomography (CT) guidance. CT guidance does not permit real-time control and precise centering is longer. However, contrast-enhanced CT shows regions of hypoattenuation devoid of characteristic parenchymal enhancement immediately after ablation, representing the areas of necrosis obtained.

In our center, the therapy plan foresees the completion of treatment in only 1 session, with an eventual retreatment after the first control of therapeutic efficacy. Because the procedure may be painful, it is performed under sedation/analgesia when 1 or 2 insertions are foreseen (in lesions <2 cm), or under general anesthesia with tracheal intubation when a greater number is planned. RFA is performed with real-time US guidance. A guide device incorporated into the US probe is used for electrode placement, permitting different angles of inclination, from 0 to 30°. After cleansing of the skin with iodized alcohol, which also serves as contact medium, the most appropriate approach for electrode insertion is selected. For lesions located in the right lobe, an intercostal approach with the patient in the left lateral decubitus position is generally preferred. For lesions located in the left lobe, a subcostal approach is used most often. The goal of therapy is to destroy the nodule and 0.5 cm of tissue surrounding it. The more the tumor increases in size, the more difficult it is to obtain a safety margin. Using the appropriate number of insertions it is not difficult to reach the complete necrosis of the nodule, even in cases larger than 5 cm, because of the so-called oven effect, which obtains large volumes of necrosis into neoplastic tissue, greater than into cirrhotic tissue. Usually we use 18-gauge internally cooled RF electrodes, single, with 2.0 or 3.0 cm of exposed metallic tip. The appearance and progression of hyperechogenicity is used to guide the duration of therapy. RF is applied until the tumor and the safety margin (when possible) surrounding it appears completely hyperechoic, and the hyperechoic focus does not increase in size for some minutes. Furthermore, in cases in which multiple insertions are required, each subsequent electrode placement is directed to an area of the tumor where hyperechogenicity is not evident. Each application of RF energy lasts 8 to 12 minutes, and in all cases the entire treatment is less than 1 hour. After therapy, patients are hospitalized for another day. Similar procedures are performed elsewhere with outpatients.

This article reports some important practical points suggested by Rhim and colleagues,[13] from one of the leading centers in this field, for obtaining a successful RF ablation, a lesson learned from 3000 procedures. We have an equivalent experience in number of patients treated, and agree with this kind of patient management. We divide Rhim and colleagues' suggestions into 3 categories: best planning, safe ablation, and complete ablation.

1. "Planning includes the following: (i) to assess feasibility of procedure based on inclusion/exclusion criteria; (ii) decision of type of approach (ie, percutaneously, laparoscopically, open), electrodes, guiding modalities and number of ablations; (iii) to decide whether to apply overlapping ablations or a special technical tip (eg, artificial ascites) for safe and complete ablation. The feasibility assessment for RFA begins with a review of good quality CT or MR [magnetic resonance] imaging. These preoperative studies are used to determine the number and size of tumors and their relationship to surrounding structures including blood vessels or vital organs. An operator should perform planning US if a US-guided procedure is considered. An operator should assess size of the tumor, whether there is a safe electrode path to the tumor, whether there is any organ close to the expected RFA zones, whether there is any large vessel close to the tumor and whether there are factors favorable for percutaneous approach. Thus, an operator should consider an alternative approach, alternative guiding modality or alternative treatment modalities (eg, PEI, PAI, TACE [transcatheter arterial chemoembolization]) depending on the degree of feasibility or the cause of technical difficulty. HCC generally requires more than a single treatment modality. Hence, we should select the proper treatment modality based on the status of the initial and recurrent tumors. Tailor-made ablation strategies with multimodality treatments may be the best approach for successful ablation outcomes."[14]

2. "Minimal invasiveness is a clear advantage of image-guided ablation over the surgical treatment. Safe ablation can be supported by careful patient selection, close patient monitoring during the ablation and appropriate management of complication after the ablation. As careful patient selection cannot guarantee safe ablation, early detection during or immediately after ablation is more important

for managing the major complications appropriately. To minimize the mortality resulting from the major complication, an interventional radiologist should be aware of the broad spectrum of complications encountered after RFA of hepatic tumors (eg, bleeding, massive infarction, extensive abscess with sepsis and thermal injury of the colon). The frequency of major complications may be correlated with both the experience and aggressiveness of an operator. If an operator has more aggressive posture for achieving complete ablation with enough ablative margin, the rate of major complication will be increased even treating technically feasible tumors. Although mild bowel edema or bile duct dilatation adjacent to the RFA zone was often seen at CT performed during or immediately after follow up, a major complication requiring specific treatment was very rare. However we recommend alternative treatment, especially for tumors broadly abutting colonic loops or major central bile ducts. All technical tips to minimize the complication should be considered if there is any possibility of complication at planning base. There are several technical tips to minimize collateral injury to vital organs including: (i) a different approach[15]; (ii) using artificial fluid[16,17]; (iii) using a balloon catheter; and (iv) pulling back or lifting the electrode.[18] Among them, artificial ascites has gained acceptance as a simple and effective technique for successful ablation."[19]

3. "Complete ablation is the last key to a successful local treatment. The ablative margin surrounding the index tumor is an established prognostic factor for local tumor control. Local tumor progression can develop at the margin of an ablation zone if the ablative margin is inadequate compared with acceptable ablative margins. So that there is enough ablative margin, three factors should be considered before or during the ablation: (i) the tumor size with 'mental' 3-D configuration; (ii) the configuration and size of the RFA zone made by a specific electrode; and (iii) the direction of the electrode path related to the tumor configuration. We believe that a complete ablation depends on achieving a symmetric ablative margin rather than simply increasing the volume of the ablation zone. Regarding the tumor configuration, 3-D measurement of the index tumor must be done accurately. An effective direction for the electrode path depending on the expected RFA zone made by a specific electrode, should be selected. Finally, targeting of the intended site of the tumors (the location determined during the planning phase) must be performed accurately because position changes of the electrode become difficult due to a poor sonic window caused by microbubbles. Hence, some experience in image-guided liver biopsy is mandatory for those involved in a RFA procedure. To solve this problem, multiple electrodes can be used, either at monopolar or bipolar modes, for achieving the desired ablative margin. Another inevitable obstacle in achieving a complete ablation is the heat-sink effect caused by abutting large vessels of more than 3 mm in diameter.[20] There are many options to deal with this technical challenge. One can choose a more aggressive posture using an intraoperative Pringle maneuver (only for metastatic deposits), or combined therapy with an ethanol injection or TACE for a perivascular tumor. At our institution, we recommend selective TACE rather RFA if more than 90° of the circumference of the central tumor abuts large vessels, especially at the hepatic hilum, because the possibility of an incomplete ablation and biliary complications are relatively high. We retrospectively assessed the morphologic pattern and exact site of local tumor progression after RFA in 86 patients who developed local tumor progression after RFA using internally-cooled electrodes. The most common pattern was the peripheral nodular type. The exact site of the local tumor progression was concordant with an insufficient ablative margin in 85%, a contiguous vessel in 42% and a subcapsular location in 50%. To sustain complete ablation for index tumor,

regular imaging follow up is essential. Most local tumor progressions are usually detected at the 3–4 month interval imaging studies, and can be treated by additional RFA. If the local tumor progression is very small or very subtle on planning US, one can use CEUS-guided procedure."[21]

Less frequently, RFA is performed using an intraoperative or a laparoscopic approach. The first is mainly performed by surgeons in patients with multiple lesions unresectable by traditional surgery or in patients with extended hepatectomy and with a central lesion in the opposite lobe.[22] The second is usually performed in patients with a difficult percutaneous approach.[23] However, in some surgical centers intraoperative RFA is preferred also in cases treatable percutaneously. In a meta-analysis, Mulier and colleagues[24] reported that RFA was performed percutaneously in 68% of cases, laparoscopically in 12%, or by laparotomy in 20%. In this meta-analysis, tumor-dependent factors with significantly minor local recurrences were small, neuroendocrine metastases, nonsubcapsular, and located away from large vessels, whereas physician-dependent favorable factors were surgical approach, vascular occlusion (in metastatic deposits), general anesthesia, a 1-cm intentional margin, and greater experience. Several factors may contribute to better results after a surgical approach. In particular, intraoperative US greatly improves spatial resolution, allows easy access to tumors located in the superior right lobe, and avoids damage by heating of adjacent organs, possible hemorrhage, or neoplastic seeding. We suggest the percutaneous route for patients who are too fragile to undergo laparotomy or for experienced operators confident enough to achieve a complete ablation. A paradoxic point of this review concerns the rate of local recurrence according to size and approach. It is not clear why in smaller lesions (<3 cm) the local recurrence rate was 16% after percutaneous approach versus 4% after surgical approach, whereas in medium-size lesions (3–5 cm, ie, those presenting fewer chances to be completely ablated), it was only 25% versus 21%, respectively.

EVALUATION OF THERAPEUTIC EFFICACY

To evaluate the therapeutic response, that is to determine whether the tumor has become completely necrotic or whether areas of neoplastic tissue are still present, a combination of investigations and serum assays for tumor markers is used. They are the same as those adopted during initial staging and controls. Because there have been many investigations and some of them are comparable, we prefer to routinely use only contrast-enhanced US (CEUS) (with SonoVue [Bracco, Milan, Italy])[25] and spiral multislice CT with the triphasic technique (4–5 mL/s, 30, 60, and 120 seconds after the injection of contrast medium). Others imaging techniques (angiography, MR, positron emission tomography) or biopsy are performed only in rare cases, if there is a doubt whether the response is partial or complete. If the areas of viable tissue are very small, beyond the present powers of resolution, they are not recognizable on the images at the end of the treatment. However, they are easily identified at follow-up if they are shown as zones of enhancement at CT (**Fig. 1**) or CEUS. The response is considered complete when CT and CEUS scans show the total disappearance of enhancement within the neoplastic tissue and when the same picture is confirmed at scans performed at successive controls. The absence of enhancement means the absence of blood flow because of necrotic and fibrotic modifications. Even with these characteristics, the necrotic area does not disappear and remains visible in place of the tumor even if reduced in size to different extents. CEUS is particularly useful during single-session treatment under general anesthesia in presence of

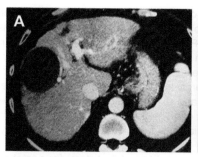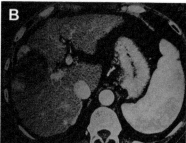

Fig. 1. (*A*) Arterial-phase CT scan obtained after RFA of a 5.9-cm HCC shows a radiologic complete necrosis (ie, no enhancement within the tumor). However, an ablative margin was not achieved. (*B*) Arterial-phase CT scan obtained 12 months after therapy shows local recurrence, because of the appearance of small peripheral nodules of extranodular growth not detectable at the baseline.

large tumors because it permits evaluation before each possible additional insertion if there is persistence of any viable area. The following energy deposition can therefore be selectively performed in the enhanced tumoral tissue.

As tumor markers, we use α-fetoprotein (AFP) and des-γ-carboxy prothrombin (DCP), which are often complementary. Nevertheless, their assay is useful only if they were abnormal before treatment. When the imaging techniques show a complete response not followed by normalization of AFP or DCP levels, it means that neoplastic tissue not detected or not yet detectable is growing elsewhere. Moreover, an increase in levels during follow-up always suggests a local recurrence or the appearance of new lesions.

We usually perform CEUS on the day after treatment, and contrast-enhanced CT if there is some doubt about ablation results. If CEUS does not present persistence of viable tissue, CT, CEUS, and serologic markers are performed every 4 months thereafter.

COMPLICATIONS

Multicenter or monocenter studies focused on complications registered mortality ranging from 0.3% to 1.4%, and a major complication rate ranging from 2.2% to 10.6%.

An Italian study reported first the complications encountered in 41 centers using percutaneous internally cooled electrodes.[26] Enrollment included 2320 patients with 3554 lesions (1610 had HCC, 693 had metastases prevalently from colorectal cancer, and 17 had cholangiocellular carcinoma). Six deaths (0.3%) were noted, including 2 caused by multiorgan failure after intestinal perforation; 1 case each of septic shock after *Staphylococcus aureus* peritonitis, massive hemorrhage after tumor rupture, liver failure after stenosis of right bile duct; and 1 case of sudden death of unknown cause 3 days after treatment. Fifty patients (2.2%) had additional major complications. The most frequent of these were peritoneal hemorrhage, neoplastic seeding, intrahepatic abscess, and intestinal perforation. All deaths occurred in patients with HCC. An increased number of RF sessions were related to a significantly higher rate of major complications.

Other studies focused on complications after RFA followed the study described earlier. De Baere and colleagues[27] performed RFA in 312 patients, using an intraoperative approach in 124 and a percutaneous approach in 226 cases. Thirty-seven

(10.6%) major complications and 5 (1.4%) deaths were reported. The deaths were by liver insufficiency in 1 case, colon perforation in 1 case, and portal vein thrombosis followed by liver insufficiency in 3 cases. Portal thrombosis was significantly more frequent in cirrhotic livers with HCC than in noncirrhotic livers after intraoperative RFA performed during a Pringle maneuver. Liver abscess was the most common major complication, occurring more frequently in patients bearing a bilioenteric anastomosis. Initially some unexpected intra- and extrahepatic complications related to the heat damage were reported in different centers (peritonitis caused by gastrointestinal tract perforation, bile duct stenosis, biliary fistulas, pleural bile lack caused by diaphragmatic injury).

Curley and colleagues[28] reported the complications of 2 centers, for a total of 608 patients with 1225 liver tumors. Open intraoperative RFA using LeVeen multiple-array electrode was performed in 382 patients, whereas percutaneous RFA was performed in 226. Mortality was 0.5% (3 cases) and early complications developed in 7.1% (43 cases), whereas late complications developed in 2.4% (15 cases). Early complications were more likely to occur after intraoperative RFA and in patients with cirrhosis. The deaths were by liver insufficiency after right lobectomy and RFA of 2 left metastases from colorectal cancer, by myocardial infarction after hypotension caused by intrahepatic bleeding in colorectal metastatic patients, and by multisystem organ failure after bacterial pneumonia in breast metastatic disease.

Kasugai and colleagues[29] reported the experience of 43 Japanese departments. Enrollment included 2542 patients with HCC. Nine deaths (0.3%) occurred, and there were 207 complications (7.9%). Deaths included 3 cases of liver failure, 3 cases of rapid progression and sarcomatous changes, 1 biliary injury, 1 gastrointestinal bleeding, and 1 acute myocardial infarction. Departments that treated larger numbers of patients per month had a smaller rate of complications.

Mulier and colleagues[30] collected all cases of complications published up to December, 2001, including some of the previous ones. Twenty cases of death were reported: 8 cases of liver failure, 6 of cardiac complications, 3 of vein thrombosis, 2 of carcinoid crisis, 1 of peritonitis, infected ascites, biliopleural fistula, hepatic abscess with diaphragmatic necrosis, hepatic abscess, chest infection, unspecified sepsis, hepatic infarction, extensive resection, extensive coagulation, peritoneal hemorrhage, and bile duct stricture.

Three types of damage were prevalently reported: thermal, septic, and mechanical. Septic and mechanical complications are in common with every percutaneous invasive procedure, such as biopsy or drainage. Thermal complications are RF related, and some of them were unexpected at the beginning of treatment. RF-related complications can be intrahepatic or extrahepatic. Intrahepatic complications are biloma, hemobilia, and stenosis caused by biliary system damage (**Fig. 2**), or thrombosis and hemorrhage caused by vascular system damage, or capsule rupture or explosive spread caused by tumoral damage. Extrahepatic complications are caused by the heat damage of organs close to the RF-treated zone, such as the gastrointestinal tract, diaphragm (**Fig. 3**), gallbladder, pleura, kidney, and skin. The following maneuvers reduce the risk of the complications discussed earlier: hot electrode withdrawal for hemorrhage, intraductal cooling for biliary stenosis, antibiotic prophylaxis for sepsis or abscesses, intraperitoneal saline infusion for detaching the liver from diaphragm or intestinal structures, PEI or selective TACE or open RFA when intraperitoneal saline infusion is not feasible because of adhesions. After the risks (some of them initially unexpected) became known, RFA became safer.

In the studies mentioned earlier, the rate of neoplastic seeding after RFA was less than 1%. However, in 2001 Llovet and colleagues[31] reported a higher and

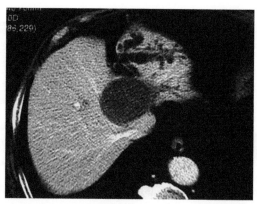

Fig. 2. CT scan obtained 4 months after therapy shows the development of marked intrahe-patic left biliary ductal dilatation distal to the zone of complete RFA tumor ablation. This asymptomatic finding did not require treatment.

unacceptable rate of 12.5% in 32 patients with HCC, finding that tumor seeding was significantly related to subcapsular location, poor degree of differentiation, and high baseline AFP levels. Subsequently Poon and colleagues[32] reported no case of seed-ing among 48 patients with subcapsular HCC and 32 patients with noncapsular HCC. Furthermore, a multicenter study focusing on this topic was published in 2005.[33] In this study a total of 1314 patients with 2542 nodules treated with the same electrode as the other studies and using the same imaging follow-up were enrolled. Neoplastic seeding was identified in 12 patients (0.9%), and the rate was comparable at the 3 centers involved. In no patient did the presence of tumor seeding have a negative effect on survival. The seeding deposits were successfully treated by surgical resection, PEI, or RFA (**Fig. 4**). Only previous diagnostic biopsy (always used with several passes in Llovet and colleagues' study), performed in 241 patients, was significantly associated with tumor seeding. Hot electrode withdrawal reduces the risk of seeding (**Fig. 5**).

Avoiding some absolute contraindications (Pringle maneuver, lesions adjacent to vital organs particularly when adhesions are suspected or to main biliary ducts,

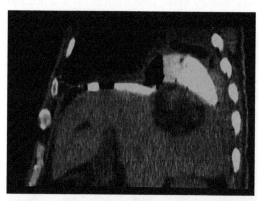

Fig. 3. CT scan with contrast media through drainage obtained some days after therapy for a 7-cm HCC shows endothoracic biloma caused by rupture of the diaphragm. The diaphrag-matic damage was probably caused by incorrect positioning of the electrode outside the tumor.

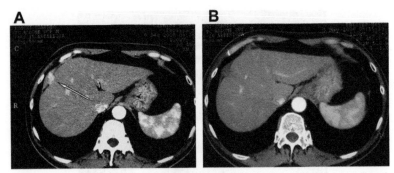

Fig. 4. (*A*) Small hypervascularized neoplastic seeding (*arrow*) detected 1 year after therapy. The patient received biopsy before RFA. (*B*) After RFA, resulted in complete ablation.

patients with bilioenteric anastomosis), RFA is a low-risk procedure. However, RFA needs adequate training because the learning curve was shown to be an independent factor in favor of adverse effects.[34]

INDICATIONS

The Barcelona Clinic Liver Cancer (BCLC) therapeutic flowchart for patients with HCC and its recommendations, because it is endorsed by the European Association for the Study of the Liver and the American Association for the Study of Liver Diseases (AASLD), are the most applied worldwide.[35] This situation means that in many centers the choice of treatment is decided according to its suggestions. This strictness is intrinsic and usual in every protocol referring to cancer treatment, but the heterogeneity of HCC presentations together with the variable score of cirrhosis should require a less defined strategy. Such recommendations involving RFA are:

a. Patients who have a single lesion can be offered surgical resection in the presence of cirrhosis but with preserved liver function, normal bilirubin and hepatic vein pressure gradient less than 10 mm Hg.
b. Liver transplantation (LT) is an effective option for patients with HCC corresponding to the Milan criteria: solitary tumor until 5 cm or up to 3 nodules less than 3 cm.

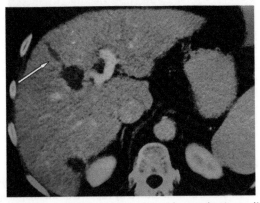

Fig. 5. Routine hot electrode withdrawal (*arrow*) avoids neoplastic seeding and reduces the risk of hemorrhage.

c. Local ablation is a safe and effective therapy for patients who cannot undergo resection, or as a bridge to transplantation. Alcohol injection and RF are equally effective for tumors less than 2 cm. However, the necrotic effect of RF is more predictable in all tumor sizes.

In recent years several referral centers, on the strength of their experience and beliefs, have proposed some changes and compared them with the BCLC/AASLD recommendations.

Stage 0 (Very Early, or Carcinoma in Situ): Single Tumor Smaller than 2 cm in Diameter, Child-Pugh Class A, Performance Status Test 0

With regard to points a and c of the BCLC/AASLD recommendations referring to the choice between hepatic resection (HR) and PAT, because of the paucity of clinical studies focused on in situ (stage 0) HCC, the literature prevalently reports those related to the treatment of single HCC less than 2 cm in diameter. In clinical practice, the very early stage is more characterized by size less than 2 cm than by its histopathologic pattern, all the more because correct diagnosis can be reached only on surgical specimens. This stage is distinguished from the early stage (stage A) because of the absence or the rarity of perinodular neoplastic invasion. Pathologic specimens describe a well-differentiated nodule with indistinct margins (the so-called indistinct type) that contains bile ducts and portal veins, to which the radiologic pattern correlates well, showing portal blood supply without tumor staining. In relation to the local invasiveness, the correct cutoff of the very early stage should have been fixed at 1.5 cm in size. Pathologists describe nodules between 1.5 and 2.0 cm (the so-called distinct type or small advanced type) containing zones of less differentiated tissue with more intense proliferative activity that give rise to portal microinvasion or microsatellites in 10% to 20% of cases (usually within 10 mm of the nodule). Increasing the diameter, the rate of microinvasion increases proportionally (ie, 30%–60% in nodules 2–5 cm and up to 60%–80% more than 5 cm).[36–42] Because no references from randomized controlled trials (RCTs) focusing on this stage have been published, we can consider 3 RCTs that compared the OS after HR and PAT (using PEI in 1 study and RFA in 2) in patients with early stage (stage A), therefore also including very early stage.[43–45] All the RCTs showed no difference in OS between the 2 groups (their results are reported in detail in the following section related to the early stage). Neither was there any statistical difference in the corresponding disease-free survival (DFS) rates. The RCTs reported shorter treatment time, less necessity for blood transfusions, lower rate of complications and shorter hospital stay in favor of PATs. Two retrospective case-control studies have been published, both using PEI.[46,47] Both reported similar OS and DFS rates, particularly when the size of single HCC was less than 3 cm (these results are reported in detail in the section related to early stage). The calculated costs per month of survival in patients treated with PEI and HR were 999 versus 3.865 euros, respectively ($P<.0001$), and hospital mortality was lower in the PEI group ($P = .055$).[46]

A cohort study conducted as a retrospective analysis of a prospective multicenter database performed on 218 patients with single HCC less than 2 cm treated with RFA was also published.[48] Two primary end points that could be easily compared with those reported for HR were assessed (ie, the rate of sustained complete response and the rate of treatment-related complications). Complete response was observed in 97.2% of patients, perioperative mortality in 0%, and major complications in 1.8%. The investigators concluded that RFA can be considered the treatment of choice even in operable patients, whereas HR can be used as salvage therapy for the few cases in which RFA is unsuccessful or unfeasible.

With regard to the comparison between PEI and RFA (in tumors <3 cm), data reported by the first controlled study on local efficacy and treatment time[49] were confirmed by the following RCTs.[50–53] They also compared local tumor progression, OS, and DFS, all presenting significantly better results in favor of RFA. Two meta-analysis studies established the same results.[54,55]

HR, when feasible, is considered the treatment of choice in patients who are not candidates for LT. This statement was not based on RCTs versus other options, but on the oncologic assumption that HR is the more suitable option for obtaining complete tumor ablation, including a layer of tissue surrounding it. This statement was established despite several non-RCTs comparing HR and PATs that failed to show better results in favor of HR. Some RCTs are now available, all revealing that OS rates in patients with early HCC are similar after PAT (principally RFA) and HR.[43–45] In very early HCC, because of the smaller tumor size, RFA should probably offer better OS because of its higher local efficacy than in early HCC. The best way to determine whether RFA is more effective than HR for very early stage is by direct comparison in an RCT. However, the results in the studies reviewed earlier indicate that the difference between the 2 approaches is small, and the sample size required to ensure meaningful results is large. For this reason a trial of this sort is probably not feasible. To give shape to such a trial a recent Markov model analysis was applied.[56] Its conclusion was that RFA followed by HR for the few cases of initial local treatment failure was nearly identical to HR regarding OS, even with the best scenario for HR and the worst scenario for RFA. Albeit under an equivalent OS, RFA offers lower complication rate, negligible perioperative mortality, lower ablation of nonneoplastic tissue, and lower costs by reducing treatment times, hospital stay, material used, and need for blood transfusions.

All the studies comparing RFA versus PEI were in favor of RFA, in terms of shortness of treatment, local efficacy, OS, and DFS, whereas the only initial advantage of PEI was the lower complication rate. When the learning curve was at an end and the risk conditions were known, the complications and mortality compared with those of PEI. However, PEI remains recommended in cases contraindicated for RFA and when RFA is not available.

Referring to points a and c of the AASLD recommendations, there are well-grounded reasons to suggest that RFA should replace HR as the therapeutic gold standard for patients with very early HCC. Furthermore, RFA is preferable to PEI also in HCC less than 2 cm because it can obtain higher local efficacy in cases presenting perinodular invasiveness.

Stage A (Early): Single Tumor or 3 Nodules Smaller than 3 cm in Diameter, Child-Pugh Class A-B, Performance Status Test 0

With regard to points a and c of the AASLD recommendations referring to the choice between HR and PAT, 5 studies have been published (3 RCTs and 2 case-control studies).[43–47]

All the RCTs reported no difference in OS and DFS rates between the 2 groups. The first trial included 76 patients with 1 or 2 nodules up to 3 cm randomly assigned to PEI or HR: the 4-year OS rates were 92% and 88%, the DFS rates 44% and 56%, and the complication rates 0% and 0%, respectively. The second trial included 161 patients with a single nodule up to 5 cm randomly assigned to RFA or HR: the 4-year OS rates were 67% and 64%, the DFS rates 46% and 51%, and perioperative mortality 0% and 3.3%, respectively. The third trial (monocenter experience partially incorporated within the previous multicenter trial) included 105 patients with a single nodule up to 5 cm or a maximum of 3 nodules up to 3 cm randomly assigned to PAT (RFA or MW ablation) or HR: the 3-year OS rates were 87% and 86%, the DFS rates 51% and 82%, and complication rates 7% and 11%, respectively. This study also compared treatment time (27 vs 145 minutes, P<.005), necessity for blood transfusion (0 vs 7 patients, P = .013), hospital stay (5 vs 19 days, P<.005), performance status test at 7 and 30 days after treatment (P = .001 and P = .004), respectively (ie, in favor of PATs). Both the case-control studies compared PEI and HR. The first included 105 carriers of a single nodule up to 5 cm: in nodules up to 3 cm the 5-year OS rates were 48% and 44%, whereas in those between 3 and 5 cm the 5-year OS rates were 17% and 54%, and DFS rates were 14% and 26%, respectively. The second study included 82 patients with a single nodule up 5 cm; the 3-year OS rates were 65% and 63%, respectively.

As reported earlier, when feasible, HR is considered the treatment of choice in patients with a single HCC who are not candidates for LT. This strategy was established despite some clinical cohort studies comparing HR and PEI that failed to show better OS in favor of HR.[57,58] In terms of OS these results were confirmed by several consequent retrospective cohort studies that on the other hand often reported a DFS significantly in favor of HR.[59–67] However, all the studies were flawed by critical drawbacks in baseline characteristics between the groups, particularly regarding the significantly better liver function for patients with HR. Because severe fibrosis is not only associated with earlier liver failure but also with a higher risk of multicentric carcinogenesis, this factor could strongly influence final outcomes. To this aim, Bruix and Sherman[35] wrote: "Theoretically, although a treatment might be less active against the tumor than another treatment and thus result in a higher recurrence rate after initial treatment, the OS might not differ or may even be better. Thus, the preferred parameter for primary comparison should be OS." Some of these studies compared OS according to the number and to the diameter of the nodules as well. Multiplicity resulted in a favorable factor for patients treated with RFA, probably because of the higher loss of nonneoplastic tissue after HR, which could anticipate the liver decompensation. After PATs, OS of patients with nodules less than 3 cm in diameter was higher than that of carriers of nodules with a diameter 3 to 5 cm, being dependent on PAT size. Why did the RCTs report that OS rates in patients with early HCC are similar after PAT (principally RFA) and HR, even with nodules greater than 3 cm? It would be reasonable to expect better OS rates among patients submitted to HR, which is seemingly the only method capable of ensuring complete ablation of nodules accompanied by peritumoral microinvasion. The equivalent outcome probably reflects the compensatory effects of certain advantages of RFA (ie, less destruction of normal tissue and lower morbidity rate), with respect to the higher local efficacy of HR.

Referring to points a and c of the AASLD recommendations, there are well-grounded reasons to suggest that RFA should be coupled with HR as the therapeutic gold standard for selected patients with early HCC (ie, with Child-Pugh class B, or with multiple tumors). With regards to size, in single nodules greater than 3 cm HR remains the first option, whereas in nodules 2 to 3 cm a peer discussion is advisable, according to individual clinical parameters (age, site, associated diseases, risk conditions) and to the operator's expertise.

With regard to RFA as a bridge to LT, this treatment is used more and more with patients on the waiting list. A critical factor determining the success of LT is the length of waiting list for a suitable donor. Llovet and colleagues[68] were the first to use an intention-to-treat principle in analyzing the outcome of patients listed for LT. Exclusion from LT as a result of tumor progression to beyond acceptable criteria and waiting list mortality are important end points in this intention-to-treat analysis. Nonresective

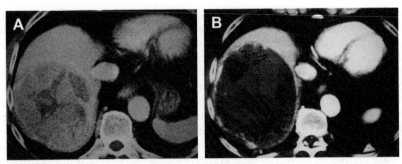

Fig. 6. (*A*) CT scan before RFA shows a huge inoperable HCC 13 cm in size occupying the right lobe. (*B*) CT scan obtained after combined therapy under general anesthesia (8 electrode insertions and PEI in some peripheral zones remained viable) shows an almost complete tumoral necrosis.

ablation, such as selective TACE or RFA, can reduce HCC progression in patients awaiting LT. A recent prospective trial had as primary end points the intention-to-treat survival, dropout, and post-LT tumor recurrence after downstaging.[69] In this study, inclusion criteria for downstaging included single nodule between 5 and 8 cm, 2 or 3 nodules with at least 1 greater than 3 cm but less than 5 cm, or 4 or 5 nodules all less than 3 cm. Criteria for successful downstaging with imaging studies included tumor size and number meeting United Network for Organ Sharing T2 criteria and complete tumor necrosis. Percutaneous RFA or PEI were prevalently used in nodules less than 4 cm, whereas TACE or laparoscopic RFA were used in bigger nodules, and these therapies were often used in combination. Tumor downstaging was successful in 70.5% of cases. In total, 57.4% of patients received LT. In the explant of 35 patients who underwent LT, 13 had complete tumor necrosis, 17 met T2 criteria, and 5 exceeded T2 criteria. The 4-year intention-to-treat survival was 92.1%, and no patient had HCC recurrence after a median post-LT follow-up of 25 months. Other studies confirmed that pre-LT therapies can significantly reduce the odds of HCC recurrence after LT and reduce HCC progression in patients on a waiting list.[70,71]

When the patient is considered inoperable, RFA can be indicated also in huge tumors, even in combination with other procedures.[14] Combination therapy with

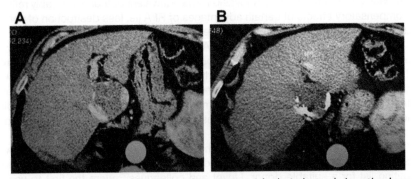

Fig. 7. (*A*) CT scan after RFA of HCC located in segment 1 (only 1 electrode insertion because of the narrow US window) shows persistence of some hypervascularized peripheral viable areas. (*B*) CT scan performed after selective TACE shows complete lipiodol uptake within viable areas.

RFA plus PEI or TACE (**Figs. 6** and **7**) can improve survival for selected patients compared with RFA alone.[72]

SUMMARY

Advances in diagnostic imaging and fine-needle biopsy techniques have permitted the development of PATs. RFA, generally performed under US guidance, is currently considered the gold standard among them. On the strength of some recent randomized trials, its indications include operable patients with small HCC, and inoperable patients with more advanced disease also in combination with other procedures. However, RFA needs adequate training because the learning curve was shown to be an independent factor in favor of adverse effects.

REFERENCES

1. Livraghi T, Festi D, Monti F, et al. US-guided percutaneous alcohol injection of small hepatic and abdominal tumors. Radiology 1986;161:309–12.
2. Masters A, Steger AC, Lees WR. Interstitial laser hyperthermia: a new approach for treating liver metastases. Br J Cancer 1992;66:518–22.
3. Rossi S, Fornari F, Buscarini L, et al. Percutaneous ultrasound guided radiofrequency electrocautery for the treatment of small hepatocellular carcinoma. J Intervent Radiol 1993;8:97–103.
4. Ohnishi K, Ohyama M, Ito S, et al. Ultrasound guided intratumor injection of acetic acid for the treatment of small hepatocellular carcinoma. Radiology 1994;193: 747–52.
5. Murakami R, Yoshimatsu S, Yamashita, et al. Treatment of hepatocellular carcinoma: value of percutaneous microwaves coagulation. Am J Roentgenol 1995; 164:1159–64.
6. Livraghi T, Vettori C, Torzilli G, et al. Percutaneous ethanol injection of hepatic tumors: single session therapy under general anesthesia. Am J Roentgenol 1993;160:1065–9.
7. Gazelle GS, Goldberg SN, Solbiati L, et al. Tumor ablation with radiofrequency energy. Radiology 2000;217:633–46.
8. McGahan PJ, Dodd DG III. Radiofrequency ablation of the liver: current status. Am J Roentgenol 2001;176:3–16.
9. Goldberg SN, Gazelle GS, Solbiati L, et al. Radiofrequency tissue ablation: increased lesion diameter with a perfusion electrode. Acad Radiol 1996;3: 636–44.
10. Goldberg SN, Solbiati L, Hahn PF, et al. Large volume tissue ablation with radiofrequency by using a clustered, internally cooled electrode technique: laboratory and clinical experience in liver metastases. Radiology 1998;209:371–9.
11. Shibata T, Shibata T, Maetani Y, et al. Radiofrequency ablation for small hepatocellular carcinoma: prospective comparison of internally cooled electrode and expandable electrode. Radiology 2006;238:346–53.
12. Lin SM, Lin CC, Chen WT, et al. Radiofrequency ablation for hepatocellular carcinoma: a prospective comparison of four radiofrequency devices. J Vasc Interv Radiol 2007;18:1118–25.
13. Rhim H, Lim HK, Kim YS, et al. Radiofrequency ablation of hepatic tumors: lessons learned from 3000 procedures. J Gastroenterol Hepatol 2008;23: 1492–500.

14. Livraghi T, Meloni F, Morabito A, et al. Multimodal image-guided tailored therapy of early and intermediate hepatocellular carcinoma: long-term survival in the experience of a single radiologic referral center. Liver Transpl 2004;10:S98–106.
15. Kim SK, Rhim H, Kim YS, et al. Radiofrequency thermal ablation of hepatic tumor: pitfalls and challenges. Abdom Imaging 2005;30:727–33.
16. Koda M, Ueki M, Maeda Y, et al. Percutaneous sonographically guided radiofrequency ablation with artificial pleural effusion for hepatocellular carcinoma located under the diaphragm. AJR Am J Roentgenol 2004;183:583–8.
17. Rhim H, Lim HK, Kim YS, et al. Percutaneous radiofrequency ablation with artificial ascites for hepatocellular carcinoma in the hepatic dome: initial experience. AJR Am J Roentgenol 2008;190:91–8.
18. Chen MH, Wei Y, Yan K, et al. Treatment strategy to optimize radiofrequency ablation for liver malignancy. J Vasc Interv Radiol 2006;17:671–83.
19. Hinshaw JL, Laeseke PF, Winter TC, et al. Radiofrequency thermal ablation of peripheral liver tumors: intraperitoneal 5% dextrose in water decrease postprocedural pain. AJR Am J Roentgenol 2006;186:S306–10.
20. Lu DS, Raman SS, Vodopich DJ, et al. Effect of vessel size on creation of hepatic radiofrequency lesions in pigs: assessment of the "heat sink" effect. AJR Am J Roentgenol 2002;1787:47–51.
21. Meloni F, Goldberg SN, Livraghi T, et al. Hepatocellular carcinoma treated with radiofrequency ablation: comparison of pulse inversion contrast-enhanced harmonic sonography, contrast-enhanced power Doppler sonography, and helical CT. AJR Am J Roentgenol 2001;177:375–80.
22. Elias D, DeBaere T, Muttillo I, et al. Intraoperative use of radiofrequency treatment allows an increase in the rate of curative liver resection. J Surg Oncol 1998;67:190–1.
23. Montorsi M, Santambrogio R, Bianchi P, et al. Radiofrequency interstitial thermal ablation of hepatocellular carcinoma in liver cirrhosis. Role of the laparoscopic approach. Surg Endosc 2001;15:141–5.
24. Mulier S, Ni Y, Jamart J, et al. Local recurrence after hepatic radiofrequency coagulation. Multivariate meta-analysis and review of contributing factors. Ann Surg 2005;242:158–71.
25. Meloni F, Livraghi T, Filice C, et al. Radiofrequency ablation of liver tumors: the role of microbubble ultrasound contrast agents. Ultrasound Q 2006;22:41–7.
26. Livraghi T, Solbiati L, Meloni F, et al. Treatment of focal liver tumors with radiofrequency ablation: complications encountered in a multicenter study. Radiology 2003;226:441–51.
27. de Baere T, Risse O, Kuoch V, et al. Adverse events during radiofrequency treatment of 582 hepatic tumors. AJR Am J Roentgenol 2003;181:695–700.
28. Curley SA, Marra P, Beaty K, et al. Early and late complications after radiofrequency ablation of malignant liver tumors in 608 patients. Ann Surg 2004;239:450–8.
29. Kasugai H, Osaki Y, Oka H, et al. Severe complications of radiofrequency ablation therapy for hepatocellular carcinoma: an analysis of 3,891 ablations in 2,614 patients. Oncology 2007;1:S72–5.
30. Mulier S, Mulier P, Ni Y, et al. Complications of radiofrequency coagulation of liver tumours. Br J Surg 2002;89:1206–22.
31. Llovet JM, Vilana R, Brù C, et al. Increased risk of tumor seeding after percutaneous radiofrequency ablation for single hepatocellular carcinoma. Hepatology 2001;33:1124–9.
32. Poon RT, Ng KK, Lam CM, et al. Radiofrequency ablation for subcapsular hepatocellular carcinoma. Ann Surg Oncol 2004;11:281–9.

33. Livraghi T, Lazzaroni S, Meloni F, et al. Risk of tumour seeding after percutaneous radiofrequency ablation for hepatocellular carcinoma. Br J Surg 2005;92:856–8.
34. Poon RT, Ng KK, Lam CM, et al. Learning curve for radiofrequency ablation of liver tumors: prospective analysis of initial 100 patients in a tertiary institution. Ann Surg 2004;239:441–9.
35. Bruix J, Sherman M. Management of hepatocellular carcinoma. Hepatology 2005; 42:1208–36.
36. Kojiro M, Nakashima O. Histopathologic evaluation of hepatocellular carcinoma with special reference to small early stage tumors. Semin Liver Dis 1999;19:287–96.
37. Kojiro M. Focus on dysplastic nodules and early hepatocellular carcinoma: an Eastern point of view. Liver Transpl 2004;10(Suppl):3A–8A.
38. Okusaka T, Okada S, Ueno H, et al. Satellite lesions in patients with small hepatocellular carcinoma with reference to clinicopathologic features. Cancer 2002; 95:1931–7.
39. Nakashima Y, Nakashima O, Tanaka M, et al. Portal vein invasion and intrahepatic micrometastasis in small hepatocellular carcinoma by gross type. Hepatol Res 2003;26:142–7.
40. Maeda T, Takenaka K, Taguchi K, et al. Small hepatocellular carcinoma with minute satellite nodules. Hepatogastroenterology 2000;47:1063–6.
41. Sasaki Y, Imaoka S, Ishiguro S, et al. Clinical features of small hepatocellular carcinomas as assessed by histologic grades. Surgery 1996;119:252–60.
42. Kanai T, Hirohashi S, Upton MP, et al. Pathology of small hepatocellular carcinoma. Cancer 1987;60:810–9.
43. Huang GT, Lee PH, Tsang YM, et al. Percutaneous ethanol injection versus surgical resection for the treatment of small hepatocellular carcinoma: a prospective study. Ann Surg 2005;242:36–42.
44. Chen MS, Li JQ, Zheng Y, et al. A prospective randomized trial comparing percutaneous local ablative therapy and partial hepatectomy for small hepatocellular carcinoma. Ann Surg 2006;243:321–8.
45. Lu MD, Kuang M, Liang LJ, et al. Surgical resection versus percutaneous thermal ablation for early-stage hepatocellular carcinoma: a randomized clinical trial. Zhonghua Yi Xue Za Zhi 2006;86:801–5.
46. Gournay J, Tchuenbou J, Richou C, et al. Percutaneous ethanol injection vs. resection in patients with small single hepatocellular carcinoma: a retrospective case-control study with cost analysis. Aliment Pharmacol Ther 2002;16:1526–38.
47. Daniele B, de Sio I, Izzo F, et al. Hepatic resection and percutaneous ethanol injection as treatments of small hepatocellular carcinoma: a CLIP retrospective case-control study. J Clin Gastroenterol 2003;36:63–7.
48. Livraghi T, Meloni F, Di Stasi M, et al. Sustained complete response and complications rates after radiofrequency ablation of very early hepatocellular carcinoma in cirrhosis: is resection still the treatment of choice? Hepatology 2008;47:82–9.
49. Livraghi T, Goldberg SN, Lazzaroni S, et al. Small hepatocellular carcinoma: treatment with radiofrequency ablation versus ethanol injection. Radiology 1999;210: 655–61.
50. Lencioni R, Allgaier HP, Cioni D, et al. Small hepatocellular carcinoma: randomized comparison of radiofrequency thermal ablation versus percutaneous ethanol injection. Radiology 2003;228:235–40.
51. Lin SM, Lin CJ, Lin CC, et al. Randomized controlled trial comparing percutaneous radiofrequency thermal ablation, percutaneous ethanol injection and percutaneous acetic acid injection to treat hepatocellular carcinoma of 3 cm or less. Gut 2005;54:1151–6.

52. Shiina S, Teratani T, Obi S, et al. A randomized controlled trial of radiofrequency ablation with ethanol injection for small hepatocellular carcinoma. Gastroenterology 2005;129:122–30.
53. Brunello F, Veltri A, Carucci P, et al. Radiofrequency ablation versus ethanol injection for early hepatocellular carcinoma: a randomized controlled study. Scand J Gastroenterol 2008;43:727–35.
54. Bouza C, Lopez-Cuadrado T, Alcazar R, et al. Meta-analysis of percutaneous radiofrequency ablation versus ethanol injection in hepatocellular carcinoma. BMC Gastroenterol 2009;9:31–40.
55. Orlando A, Leandro G, Olivo M, et al. Radiofrequency thermal ablation vs percutaneous ethanol injection for small hepatocellular carcinoma: meta-analysis of randomized controlled trials. Am J Gastroenterol 2009;104:514–24.
56. Cho YK, Kim JK, Kim WT, et al. Hepatic resection versus radiofrequency ablation for very early stage hepatocellular carcinoma: a Markov model analysis. Hepatology 2010;51:1–7.
57. Livraghi T, Bolondi L, Buscarini L, et al. No treatment, resection and ethanol injection in hepatocellular carcinoma: a retrospective analysis of survival in 391 patients with cirrhosis. J Hepatol 1995;22:522–6.
58. Ryu M, Shimamura Y, Kinoshita T, et al. Therapeutic results of resection, transcatheter arterial embolization and percutaneous ethanol injection in 3225 patients with hepatocellular carcinoma: a retrospective multicenter study. Jpn J Clin Oncol 1997;27:251–7.
59. Cho CM, Tak WY, Kweon YO, et al. [The comparative results of radiofrequency ablation versus surgical resection for the treatment of hepatocellular carcinoma]. Korean J Hepatol 2005;11:59–71 [in Korean].
60. Hong SN, Lee SY, Choi MS, et al. Comparing the outcomes of radiofrequency ablation and surgery in patients with a single small hepatocellular carcinoma and well-preserved hepatic function. J Clin Gastroenterol 2005; 39:247–52.
61. Ogihara M, Wong LL, Machi J. Radiofrequency ablation versus surgical resection for single nodule hepatocellular carcinoma: long-term results. HPB (Oxford) 2005;7:214–21.
62. Wakai T, Shirai Y, Suda T, et al. Long-term outcomes of hepatectomy vs percutaneous ablation for treatment of hepatocellular carcinoma. World J Gastroenterol 2006;12:546–52.
63. Takahashi S, Kudo M, Chung H, et al. Outcomes of nontransplant potentially curative therapy for early stage hepatocellular carcinoma in Child-Pugh stage A cirrhosis is comparable with liver transplantation. Dig Dis 2007;25:303–9.
64. Hasegawa K, Makuuchi M, Takayama T, et al. Surgical resection vs percutaneous ablation for hepatocellular carcinoma: a preliminary report of the Japanese nationwide survey. J Hepatol 2008;49:589–94.
65. Nanashima A, Masuda J, Miuma S, et al. Selection of treatment modality for hepatocellular carcinoma according to the modified Japan Integrated Staging score. World J Gastroenterol 2008;14:58–63.
66. Abu-Hilal M, Primrose JN, Casaril A, et al. Surgical resection versus radiofrequency ablation in the treatment of small unifocal hepatocellular carcinoma. J Gastrointest Surg 2008;12:1521–6.
67. Ueno S, Sakoda M, Kubo F, et al. Surgical resection versus radiofrequency ablation for small hepatocellular carcinomas within the Milan criteria. J Hepatobiliary Pancreat Surg 2009;16:359–66.

68. Llovet JM, Fuster J, Bruix J. Intention-to-treat analysis of surgical treatment for early hepatocellular carcinoma. Hepatology 1999;30:1434–40.
69. Yao FY, Kerlan RK, Hirose R, et al. Excellent outcome following down-staging of hepatocellular carcinoma prior to liver transplantation: an intention-to-treat analysis. Hepatology 2008;48:819–27.
70. Maluf D, Fisher RA, Maroney T, et al. Non-resective ablation and liver transplantation in patients with cirrhosis and hepatocellular carcinoma: safety and efficacy. Am J Transplant 2003;3:312–7.
71. Lao OB, Weissman J, Perkins JD. Pre-transplant therapy for hepatocellular carcinoma is associated with a lower recurrence after liver transplantation. Clin Transplant 2009;23:874–81.
72. Cabibbo, Latteri F, Antonucci, et al. Multimodal approaches to the treatment of hepatocellular carcinoma. Nat Clin Pract Gastroenterol Hepatol 2009;6:159–69.

Planning and Follow-up After Ablation of Hepatic Tumors: Imaging Evaluation

Piyaporn Boonsirikamchai, MD, Evelyne M. Loyer, MD,
Haesun Choi, MD, Chusilp Charnsangavej, MD*

KEYWORDS

- Liver tumor • Radiofrequency ablation
- Computed tomography • Magnetic resonance imaging

Over the past two decades, radiofrequency ablation (RFA) has been used increasingly to treat both resectable and unresectable hepatic tumors, in particular early-stage hepatocellular carcinoma (HCC) and unresectable colorectal hepatic metastases (CRHMs). Consequently, the efficacy of RFA in treatment of hepatic tumors has been thoroughly studied and reviewed but has varied from study to study. Recently, the American Society of Clinical Oncology conducted a large systemic review that showed the wide variability of the reported 5-year survival rate (14% to 55%) and local tumor recurrence rate (3.6% to 60%) of patients who underwent RFA for unresectable CRHM.[1] This variability is partly due to the difference in patient or tumor selection criteria, tumor biology, or technical experience.[1]

Imaging studies play an important role in tumor staging and help select good candidates for ablation, which leads to successful performance of RFA. Moreover, imaging studies help assess treatment success, identify incomplete ablation or residual tumor that needs further treatment or additional ablation, and identify complications after ablation. Eradication of residual tumors at early stage and appropriate management of complications may increase disease-free survival and overall survival of patients after RFA.

There are various imaging modalities used for tumor staging and treatment assessment of RFA. CT and MRI are the modalities of choice for tumor staging and follow-up after RFA. MRI has better soft tissue contrast and, therefore, is superior to CT in sensitivity to detect small lesion (<1 cm). CT is more frequently used, however, because of

Piyaporn Boonsirikamchai: research fellow in Diagnostic Radiology, partly supported by the Robert D. Moreton Distinguished Chair in Diagnostic Radiology. Chusilp Charnsangavej: consultant, Novartis Pharmaceuticals Inc.

Department of Diagnostic Radiology, The University of Texas MD Anderson Cancer Center, Unit 1473, PO Box 301402, Houston, TX 77230-1402, USA

* Corresponding author.

E-mail address: ccharn@mdanderson.org

Surg Oncol Clin N Am 20 (2011) 301–315
doi:10.1016/j.soc.2010.11.007
1055-3207/11/$ – see front matter © 2011 Elsevier Inc. All rights reserved.

its greater availability. Contrast-enhanced ultrasound with microbubble contrast agent, with experienced operators, has been shown to have diagnosis accuracy comparable to CT or MRI[2]; however, it is not widely applicable.[3,4] Availability of micro-bubble contrast agent and being operator-dependent are significant limitations of ultrasound. Combined positron emission tomography and CT (PET/CT) has demon-strated good sensitivity in detection of early tumor recurrence after RFA; thus, it may be used as a problem-solving tool.[5–7] PET/CT has no potential role in HCC, however, because HCC is often PET negative.

This article reviews the current roles of imaging studies, focusing on CT and MRI, in planning and follow-up of hepatic tumors after ablation. Tumor selection, immediate treatment assessment, subsequent and long-term follow-up, and pattern of local tumor progression as well as immediate and delayed complications of RFA are described.

PRETREATMENT IMAGING

Optimal imaging technique and spatial resolution provide good anatomic detail, which is required to make decisions on patient management. A large review study has shown that 52% of patients with CRHMs who were referred to a tertiary care center had inad-equate imaging at the time of referral, and additional imaging studies changed the expected management in 30% of these patients.[1]

Generally, a multidetector CT scanner and multiphasic contrast enhancement are required for detection and characterization of hypervascular hepatic tumors and preoperative or preablative planning. HCC and hypervascular metastases, such as neuroendocrine carcinoma, renal cell carcinoma, and breast cancer, characteristically appear as a transiently hyperattenuating mass during the hepatic arterial phase and become isoattenuating or hypoattenuating with liver parenchyma in the portal venous phase of enhancement. Alternatively, hypovascular tumors, such as metastases from colorectal cancer, usually appear as hypoattenuating mass in the portal venous phase.

On MRI, HCC and metastases usually are hypointense on T1-weighted images and hyperintense on T2-weighted images. HCC, however, may be isointense or hyperin-tense on T1-weighted images. The MRI patterns of enhancement of HCC and metas-tases are similar to CT.

The important factors that have an impact on the successful rate of RFA include tumor appearance, size, number, location, and invasion of adjacent structures or organs.

Size and Numbers

For HCC, patients are required to have a single tumor smaller than 5 cm or as many as three nodules smaller than 3 cm each.[8]

For hepatic metastases, there is no clear consensus regarding the size and number of lesions that should be treated with RFA. The highest ablation success rates, however, have been achieved in patients with a solitary CRHM or a few CRHMs less than 3 cm in diameter.[9–11] Although larger tumors can be treated by overlapping ablations, the chance of incomplete ablation seems to increase as the size of tumors increase (**Fig. 1**).[12] In many studies, the local recurrence rate for tumors larger than 5 cm is significantly greater than for tumors between 3 and 5 cm.[13,14]

Location

Multiple studies have reported an increased failure rate in tumors adjacent to large blood vessels (diameter >1 cm).[14–16] Large blood vessels tend to be protected by

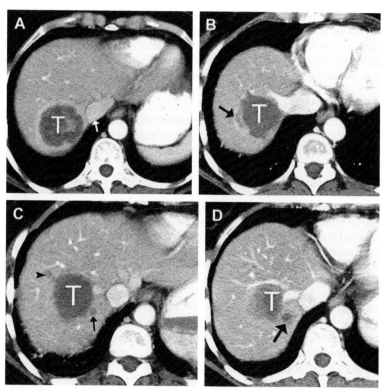

Fig. 1. RFA of large metastatic colorectal carcinoma to the liver with recurrent tumor at the periphery of the ablation zone. (*A*) Pretreatment CT showed a 5-cm metastasis (T) in segment VII adjacent to the inferior vena cava (*arrow*). (*B*) One month after ablation, the tumor (T) became necrotic showing hypodensity change without enhancement. Note enhancement (*arrow*) at the periphery of the ablated zone suspicious for tumor recurrence. (*C*) The scan 2 cm below the level (*B*), however, defined a small nodule (*arrow*) posterior to the ablated zone (T). Also note the tract (*arrowhead*) from RFA. (*D*) Three months later, recurrent tumor (*arrow*) became more apparent at the periphery of the ablated lesion (T).

the intrinsic cooling provided by the blood flowing through them, the so-called heat-sink effect.[17] Blood flow can negatively affect the results of RFA because it can potentially remove heat before complete tumor ablation is achieved.[8]

The location of a tumor not only affects the successful rate of RFA but may also affect the complication rate. Ablation of tumors located near the portal vein pedicles is associated with major bile duct injury, resulting in biliary stricture and sepsis.[1] Tumors at subcapsular location are more challenging to treat percutaneously because of the risk of thermal injury to adjacent organs, such as the diaphragm and the bowel loop. In such instances, the use of special techniques, such as intraperitoneal injection of dextrose to displace the bowel, can be considered.[8]

Bile Duct or Major Vessel Invasion

Bile duct and major vessel invasion are usually contraindications for RFA. Contrast-enhanced CT and MRI are capable of demonstrating vascular invasion in HCC. Tumor thrombus usually appears as an intravascular filling defect with streaky or homogeneous enhancement, which helps distinguish it from bland thrombus that does not show enhancement. HCC may also cause biliary ductal dilatation by compression or, less commonly, by direct intraductal invasion. Similarly, metastases, particularly from colorectal cancer, may invade adjacent bile duct.[18] Careful review imaging is necessary to detect subtle tumor thrombus or bile duct invasion.

Extrahepatic Metastases

Extrahepatic metastases are usually a contraindication for RFA. They are occasional exceptions, however, in patients treated with effective chemotherapy with residual liver-only metastases or in patients with lung metastases that can be resected.[19]

TREATMENT ASSESSMENT

Currently, there is no consensus on a standard follow-up interval regimen for imaging. The most common approach by members of the International Working Group on Image-Guided Tumor Ablation includes contrast-enhanced CT or MRI within 6 weeks of the initial ablation to determine whether or not additional ablation therapy is required and every 3 to 4 months thereafter to determine technique effectiveness.[20]

Imaging with intravenous contrast is needed because pathologic studies have shown that the best correlation of necrotic tissue is defined by the zone of nonenhancement on cross-sectional studies.[21–23] Patients who have undergone RFA for hypervascular tumors, such as HCC, need to be evaluated before and after intravenous administration of a contrast agent with a protocol that includes image acquisition during the arterial phase of enhancement. Small hypervascular tumor nodules could be overlooked if this phase is not performed.

Immediate Follow-up

Complete ablation

On noncontrast CT, the ablative zone appears as a sharply demarcated low attenuation but often contains area of high attenuation along the electrode needle tract or in the center.[21] This high attenuation area is thought to represent greater cellular disruption and it should resolve in the successive weeks or months.[21] Air bubbles produced during ablation may be seen at immediate follow-up and usually resolve within 1 month.[24] The shape of ablation zone is usually round or oval, depending on the electrode type used in the procedure.[25–27] The shape may be irregular, however, when the index tumor is located between large branches of hepatic vessels where there is heat sink effect from blood flow.[24]

After contrast administration, the ablative zone typically appears as a nonenhancing area of low attenuation, representing coagulative necrosis (**Figs. 1** and **2**). The most important morphologic features of complete ablation are the size and the characteristic smooth margin of the ablative zone.[25] The ablative zone should be larger than the index tumor, centered at the index tumor, and encompass the entire index tumor[28] with an additional circumferential ablative margin, ideally 0.5 to 1.0 cm in thickness.[8] The ablative margin is the region of ablated hepatic parenchyma beyond the border of tumor that assures the destruction of locally invasive microscopic tumor.[8] The interface between the ablative lesion and adjacent normal hepatic parenchyama should be sharply demarcated.

Benign periablational enhancement is frequently seen in immediate follow-up study and usually disappears by the time of a 1-month follow-up examination[27]; however, it can last up to 6 months.[29] In pathologic specimens, this benign peripheral enhancement has been shown to be a peripheral zone of congestion and sinusoidal

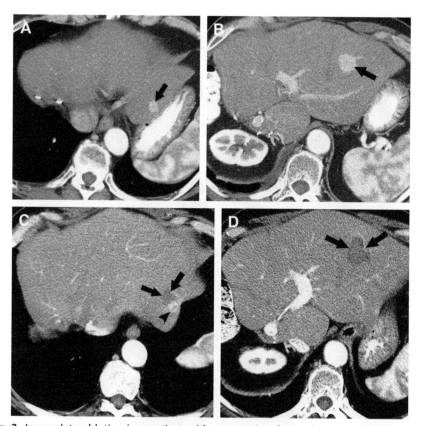

Fig. 2. Incomplete ablation in a patient with metastatic colorectal cancer to the liver and had prior right liver resection. (*A*) CT of the abdomen during arterial phase demonstrated a small hyperdense enhancing tumor (*arrow*) near the posterior surface of segment II. (*B*) Another tumor (*arrow*) was identified between segment II and III. (*C*) Three months after RFA, the lesion near the posterior surface of segment II was not completely ablated. Note the hyperdense enhancing nodule (*arrowhead*) posterior to the hypodense ablated zone (*arrows*). (*D*) The tumor between segment II and III was completely ablated and appeared hypodense (*arrows*). Repeated ablation of the lesion near the posterior surface of segment II was performed.

hemorrhage, gradually replaced by granulation tissue.[21] This benign periablational enhancement is most appreciated on the arterial phase of CT scan and variable in intensity and thickness depending on the scanning technique. It is concentric, symmetric, and uniform in appearance with smooth inner margins and must be differentiated from irregular or nodular peripheral enhancement seen in incomplete ablation.[20] Benign wedge-shaped enhancement at or distal to the ablation zone may be seen in arterial phase due to a compensatory increase in arterial flow in a territory where portal branches have been destroyed.

The morphologic characteristics of the ablation zone on CT can also be applied to MRI. Specific to MRI are changes in signal intensity. The ablative zone has variable signal intensity on T1-weighted images. Complete ablation is characterized by low signal intensity on T2-weighted images (**Fig. 3**), whereas a viable tumor produces

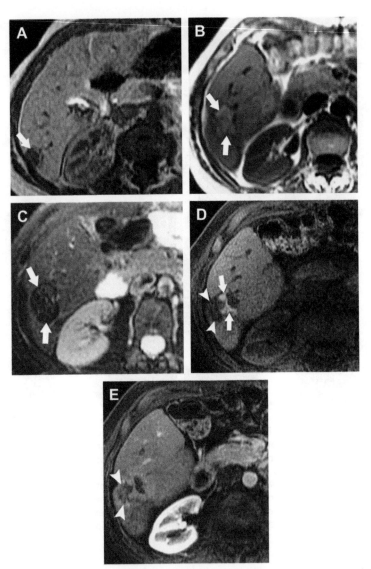

Fig. 3. MRI appearances of postablation therapy and recurrent tumor in a patient with hepatic metastasis from colorectal cancer. (*A*) T1-weighted axial image of the liver showed a hypointense, metastatic tumor (*arrow*) at the periphery of segment VI. (*B*) Six months after ablation therapy, the zone of ablation therapy (*arrows*) became hyperintense relative to the surrounding hepatic parenchyma on this T1-weighted image. (*C*) T2-weighted image showed the hypointense ablated zone (*arrows*). (*D*) Two years later, the hyperintense ablated zone (*arrows*) became contracted but hypointense region (*arrowheads*) was identified at the periphery of the ablated zone on this T1-weighted axial image. (*E*) Postgadolinium, contrast-enhanced, T1-weighted image defined the enhancing nodule (*arrowheads*) at the periphery of the ablated zone and was histologically confirmed as recurrent tumor.

high signal intensity.[30] In the first week after ablation, however, T2 signal intensity can also be variable depending on the stage of hemorrhage and liquefactive or coagulative necrosis.[31,32] Therefore, to maximize the accuracy of the study, contrast administration with gadolinium is routinely used. Similar to CT, benign periablational enhancement is often seen as an ill-defined perilesional rim with high signal intensity on T2-weighted images and moderate to intense enhancement on arterial dominant-phase images. Lack of nodular or irregular enhancement indicates complete ablation.[31,32]

On immediate follow-up studies, differentiation of benign periablational enhancement from residual tumor may be difficult. If the findings on cross-sectional images are inconclusive, PET/CT may be useful as problem-solving in cases of hepatic metastases (Fig. 4).[5–7] For HCC cases, close follow-up with CT or MRI is necessary.

Incomplete ablation

On immediate follow-up, incomplete ablation with residual tumor is always suspected if the ablation zone does not cover the entire index tumor.[24] Residual unablated tumor can be mostly identified at the periphery of the ablation zone and may be subtle.[25]

Residual unablated hypervascular tumor usually appears as a nodular or asymmetric enhancing area at the margin of the ablation zone (see **Figs. 2** and **3**). This enhancement may sometimes be seen only during the arterial phase, emphasizing the importance of the scan technique.[33] For an index tumor with hypovascularity, the residual tumor may appear as a disruption of the smooth interface between the ablation zone and the surrounding hepatic parenchyma.[24] This observation may be difficult to identify because of the benign periablational enhancement that is often seen on immediate follow-up of cross-sectional images.[24] Eccentric and focal areas of enhancement are more likely indicative of residual tumor tissue than of a benign cause of enhancement (see **Fig. 3**).[20,27]

On MRI, the residual tumor may appear as a nodule distorting the internal contour of the ablation zone and typically shows moderately high signal intensity on T2-weighted images with peripheral nodular or irregular enhancement on arterial dominant-phase that may persist on late-phase images (see **Fig. 3**).[31,34]

Subsequent and Long-Term Follow-up

Complete ablation

The ablation zone becomes better circumscribed when compared to immediate follow-up images and typically involutes gradually. Volume changes compared with the volume at the immediate follow-up CT examination have been reported as 79%,

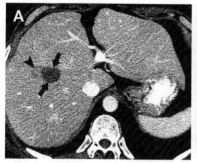 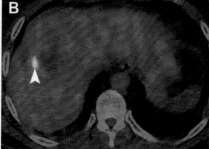

Fig. 4. Recurrent tumor after RFA demonstrated on CT and PET/CT. (*A*) Axial CT image illustrated a hypodense, postablation, lesion (*arrows*) with a nodule (*arrowhead*) at the periphery. (*B*) PET/CT image demonstrated a high glucose uptake of the nodule (*arrowhead*) at the periphery of the treated lesion, confirmed as a recurrent tumor.

50%, 27%, 11%, and 6% at 1, 4, 10, 16, and 19 months, respectively.[27] The rate of involution, however, can be varied from case to case and no or minimal involution does not always imply treatment failure. No or minimal involution may be due to the complication of RFA, such as biloma formation or abscess.[20]

As discussed previously, benign periablational enhancement, which is seen in immediate follow-up, usually disappears by the time of a 1-month follow-up. On CT, the ablation zone usually appears as a well-circumscribed hypoattenuating area without enhancement. On MRI, the ablation zone shows more homogeneous signal intensity with hyperintensity on T1-weighted and hypointensity on T2-weighted images.

Local tumor progression

The term, *local tumor progression*, indicates both incompletely treated viable tumor that was previously considered completely treated but continued to grow and a new tumor, such as satellite or daughter lesions of HCC, that grows at the original site. Local tumor progression may be subtle and most often occurs at the periphery of the ablated lesion.[20]

Local tumor progression can be classified into three patterns.[35] First, the nodular type appears as focal nodule enhancement at the margin of the ablation zone. It may be a small nodule with only slightly higher attenuation than necrotic tissues that protrude within the defect or a faint hypoattenuating zone that extends into the adjacent parenchyma.[25] Second, the halo type appears as rim enhancement at the margin of the ablation zone.[20] The third pattern is gross enlargement pattern that shows an increase in overall tumor size.[29,35]

On MRI, pattern of local tumor progression is similar to CT. Local tumor progression usually appears as a development of T1-hypointense and T2-hyperintense signal areas with irregular or nodular enhancement.

New hepatic lesion and extrahepatic disease

New hepatic lesions and extrahepatic disease are the majority of recurrence, with a rate of 47% compared with 9% for local recurrence.[36] Careful evaluation of follow-up CT or MRI is essential to detect new hepatic metastases outside the ablation zone (**Fig. 5**) and extrahepatic lesions.

COMPLICATIONS

RFA is a relatively safe procedure with a low mortality rate (0%–2%)[1] and low major complication rate (2.2%–3.1%).[8] The major complications include intraperitoneal bleeding, liver abscess, intestinal perforation, pneumothorax and hemothorax, bile duct stenosis, and tumor seeding.[8] The most common complications are intraperitoneal bleeding, hepatic abscess, bile duct injury, hepatic decompensation, and grounding pad burns, whereas the most common causes of death are sepsis, hepatic failure, colon perforation, and portal vein thrombosis. Complications may be early, occurring in the first 30 days after RFA, or delayed, occurring after 30 days.[1] Vascular injury and injury to adjacent organs are usually detected early after RFA,[37,38] whereas tumor seeding is usually detected at long-term follow-up.[37] Abscess and biliary complication can be either immediate or delayed complication. Early detection and accurate evaluation are essential for the proper management of the complications.

Immediate Complications

Vascular complications

Vascular complications may be mechanical injuries caused by the radiofrequency electrode traversing a vessel or thermal injury sustained during ablation.[39] Arterial

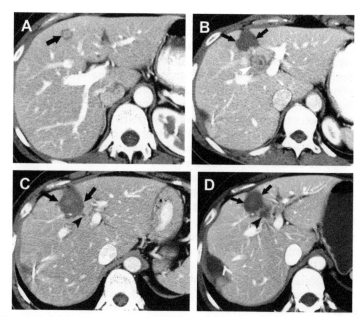

Fig. 5. Metastatic leiomyosarcoma to the liver treated with resection and RFA. (*A*) Axial CT image demonstrated a metastatic lesion (*arrow*) near the anterior surface of segment IV. Another lesion in the right liver under the diaphragm was not shown but was also treated. (*B*) Fifteen months after RFA, the treated lesion remained hypodense (*arrows*). New lesion (*arrowhead*) was found, however, near the posterior surface of segment IV adjacent to the bile duct and the bifurcation of the portal vein in the hilar fissure. (*C*) Repeated ablation was performed and the ablated zone (*arrows*) was expanded. Small residual nodule (*black arrowhead*) was noted on the image. (*D*) Two years later, recurrent tumor (*black arrowhead*) was discovered posterior to the ablated zone (*arrows*). Recurrent tumor was also discovered in the treated lesion at the right liver under the diaphragm (not entirely shown).

bleeding, pseudoaneurysm, arteriovenous fistula, and hepatic vein thrombosis (HVT) and portal vein thrombosis (PVT) have been reported.

Intraperitoneal bleeding

Coagulopathy is the most important risk factor for bleeding after RFA. Thus, patients with cirrhosis are considered at higher risk than those without cirrhosis.[37] Other risk factors include the use of multiple punctures or multiple electrodes and the location of the targeted lesion behind a major blood vessel.[37]

If bleeding is suspected, CT is the modality of choice for the detection and evaluation of hematoma.[37] Bleeding usually appears as high-attenuation fluid surrounding the liver and may extend into the adjacent extraperitoneal space. Transfusion is required in patients who develop severe anemia. Although most of post-RFA bleeding stops spontaneously, transcatheter arterial embolization is uncommonly required, particularly when the bleeding is from an artery.[37]

Pseudoaneurysm

A pseudoaneurysm of the intrahepatic artery is rare. It may appear as a small, intense, nodular enhancement lesion at the ablation zone. Because it can be small, careful review of the follow-up imaging is necessary.[40]

Portal vein thrombosis and hepatic vein thrombosis

When PVT or HVT occurs as a complication of RFA, it usually manifests early after the procedure. Small vessels (<3 mm) are prone to thrombosis caused by thermal damage because vascular perfusion–mediated heat-sink effect depends on the size of the vessel.[17] Besides vessel size, amount of blood flow in the vessel also affects the heat-sink effect. Thermal damage may cause thrombosis even in large vessels if the blood flow is decreased, as happens during the Pringle maneuver (clamping the porta hepatis, which interrupts hepatic arterial and portal venous flow to the liver),[41–43] especially in cirrhotic livers.[44] Other conditions that can decrease blood flow (eg, pre-existing thrombus, previous intervention, and mechanical damage of vessels by electrode) also may be considered risk factors for PVT.[37]

On contrast-enhanced CT, thrombus appears as a filling defect in the portal vein. Segmental enhancement of the liver parenchyma peripheral to the affected portal vein is an indirect sign of thrombosis that may be observed during the hepatic arterial phase.[37] For HVT, loss of enhancement of hepatic vein during portal venous phase may be seen; however, evaluation tends to be difficult because of a delay and decrease in enhancement caused by congestion.[37] A comparison of images acquired before and after RFA may be helpful. A wedge-shaped area of decreased enhancement on hepatic arterial phase represents congestion and may be observed on the hepatic arterial phase image. Most PVTs and HVTs are self-limited; treatment may be required if liver function is affected.[37]

Hepatic infarction

Hepatic parenchymal infarction is an uncommon complication of RFA (0.7%–1.8%).[45] The major clinical symptom of hepatic infarction is pain.[46] Imaging findings show a newly developed, well-defined, wedge-shaped, nonenhancing area of low attenuation peripheral to the ablation zone.[46] Branching area of air density, probably segment of the portal veins, is frequently observed in the infarcted area.[37] The lesion undergoes slow and progressive shrinkage.[45] Management is conservative and may include the prophylactic use of antibiotics.[37]

Injury to adjacent organs

Injury to the gastrointestinal tract Early detection is essential for the management of injury to the gastrointestinal tract. RFA of a lesion adjacent to the bowel loop and adhesions caused by prior surgery or RFA can be potential risk factors of bowel injury.[37] The colon is considered a higher risk for thermal damage than are the stomach and small bowel, because of its lesser mobility and thinner wall thickness.[47]

Imaging findings show a thickened wall of the gastrointestinal tract and fat stranding around the injured site. Free air and/or ascites may be seen. Bowel injury occasionally causes an abscess in the liver or outside it. Therefore, if abscess formation is observed after RFA, close attention should be paid to the gastrointestinal tract.[37]

Injury to the gallbladder Cholecystitis may occur after RFA, but perforation of the gallbladder is rare even if the lesion treated with ablation is adjacent to the gallbladder.[48] Adhesion due to prior surgery or percutaneous therapy may be a potential risk factor for injury to the gallbladder.[37] Thickening of the gallbladder wall and surrounding fat stranding are signs of cholecystitis.[37] Perforation of the gallbladder may be associated with other complications, such as injury to the colon, and gas in the biliary system may be an indication of this type of gallbladder injury.[37] Management of perforation of the gallbladder requires percutaneous or endoscopic drainage.[37]

Pneumothorax and hemothorax

Pneumothorax and hemothorax, which are related to the image-guided placement of electrodes, are rare but may be encountered if the treated lesion is near the diaphragm.[37] Chest radiography is required if chest pain or dyspnea occurs after RFA. Lung window display is necessary for proper viewing of follow-up CT scans. Pneumothorax and hemothorax are usually self-limited.[37]

Abscess

Abscess is one of the most common major complications after RFA of the liver, with a reported incidence of 0.3% to 2.0%.[44,47,49] Abscess usually develops 2 to 8 weeks after the procedure.[38] Two important risk factors for abscess formation are recognized: bacterial colonization of the biliary tract and diabetes mellitus.[38]

US images show coarse clumps of debris and echogenicity of gas in the abscess. On nonenhanced CT, abscess appears as a hypoattenuating lesion containing gas. A double-target sign may be observed on contrast-enhanced CT.[50] As discussed previously, gas can be seen inside the ablation zone on CT scans obtained immediately after RFA but should disappear by the 1-month follow-up CT examination, if the lesion is not infected. The diagnosis of hepatic abscess, therefore, should be based both on imaging findings and on clinical symptoms, such as fever and pain.[37] Fever due to postablation syndrome is not uncommon and is usually low grade.[38] Persistent fever after 2 to 3 weeks should raise suspicion for infection.[38]

Pseudoaneurysm formation, a rare complication of hepatic abscess, may complicate the clinical course.[51] Management of hepatic abscess is based on appropriate antibiotics and percutaneous drainage.[37]

Delayed Complication

Biliary complication

Bile duct stricture The prevalence of bile duct dilatation has been reported as high as 18%.[52] Small intrahepatic bile duct dilatation peripheral to the ablation zone is presumably associated with thermal injury–induced stricture and is usually asymptomatic.[46] It begins to be noticed after several months and slowly progresses. It sometimes induces atrophic changes of the involved parenchyma similar to those seen associated with intrahepatic duct stone after years of follow-up. Even though the injury of major bile ducts near the hepatic hilum is uncommon because of the protection from the heat sink effect of the portal vein,[53,54] it sometimes occurs and needs percutaneous transhepatic biliary drainage.[46]

Biloma Biloma is formed by leakage of fluid from the injured biliary duct and mostly is asymptomatic.[46] On CT, biloma manifests as round or oval fluid collection at the ablation zone and, thus, could mimic the ablation zone itself (**Fig. 6**).[46] Biloma may increase in size slowly as seen on follow-up imaging and is often a mere fluid collection. Biloma, however, frequently contains ablated necrotic parenchyma on its inner wall as a mural nodule of cystic neoplasm.[46] If biloma causes a mass symptom, interventional drainage may be needed.[37,52]

Hemobilia Hemobilia is a rare complication and its incidence has been reported as 0.25%.[39] Melena and upper abdominal pain are the most common symptoms of hemobilia.[37]

Hemobilia appears as high-attenuation in the dilated bile duct and/or gallbladder as seen on noncontrast CT images immediately after the RFA.[55] Heterogeneous hyperechoic clots are observed in gallbladder on ultrasound images. No treatment is need in asymptomatic patients.

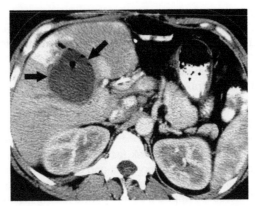

Fig. 6. Infected biloma (*arrows*) in a patient who had RFA for metastatic colorectal cancer previously treated in intra-arterial chemotherapy via an infusion port. Patients with intra-arterial chemotherapy may have an increased risk of biloma because of potential sclerosing cholangitis associated with intra-arterial chemotherapy.

Tumor seeding

Tumor seeding is a significant complication with the reported incidence 0.2% to 1.4% in HCC.[47,56,57] Tumors seeding usually occurs 3 to 12 months after RFA and can occur along the needle tract, pleural, and peritoneum depending on tumor location.[38] Caliber and type of electrode used, numbers of punctures, subcapsular location of the tumor, and poor differentiation of the tumor have been associated with needle track seeding.[58,59]

On contrast-enhanced cross-sectional imaging, tumor seeding appears as a nodular or flat lesion with early enhancement, in cases of HCC, or small hypoattenuating lesion, in cases of metastases, along the electrode tract or at the gravity-dependent position.[37] Seeded tumors occasionally grow slowly; thus, a long follow-up period is necessary to exclude tumor seeding.[37]

SUMMARY

Imaging studies play an important role in planning ablation therapy and postablation follow-up. Careful assessment of imaging studies before therapy can identify proper candidates for treatment and minimize complications. Appropriate studies after therapy can modify treatment planning and have potential to improve outcome of treatment.

REFERENCES

1. Wong SL, Mangu PB, Choti MA, et al. American Society of Clinical Oncology 2009 clinical evidence review on radiofrequency ablation of hepatic metastases from colorectal cancer. J Clin Oncol 2010;28:493–508.
2. Choi D, Lim HK, Lee WJ, et al. Early assessment of the therapeutic response to radio frequency ablation for hepatocellular carcinoma: utility of gray scale harmonic ultrasonography with a microbubble contrast agent. J Ultrasound Med 2003;22:1163–72.
3. Dill-Macky MJ, Asch M, Burns P, et al. Radiofrequency ablation of hepatocellular carcinoma: predicting success using contrast-enhanced sonography. AJR Am J Roentgenol 2006;186(Suppl):S287–95.

4. Lu MD, Yu XL, Li AH, et al. Comparison of contrast enhanced ultrasound and contrast enhanced CT or MRI in monitoring percutaneous thermal ablation procedure in patients with hepatocellular carcinoma: a multi-center study in China. Ultrasound Med Biol 2007;33:1736–49.

5. Anderson GS, Brinkmann F, Soulen MC, et al. FDG positron emission tomography in the surveillance of hepatic tumors treated with radiofrequency ablation. Clin Nucl Med 2003;28:192–7.

6. Donckier V, Van Laethem JL, Goldman S, et al. [F-18] fluorodeoxyglucose positron emission tomography as a tool for early recognition of incomplete tumor destruction after radiofrequency ablation for liver metastases. J Surg Oncol 2003;84:215–23.

7. Kuehl H, Antoch G, Stergar H, et al. Comparison of FDG-PET, PET/CT and MRI for follow-up of colorectal liver metastases treated with radiofrequency ablation: initial results. Eur J Radiol 2008;67:362–71.

8. Crocetti L, de Baere T, Lencioni R. Quality improvement guidelines for radiofrequency ablation of liver tumours. Cardiovasc Intervent Radiol 2010;33:11–7.

9. de Meijer VE, Verhoef C, Kuiper JW, et al. Radiofrequency ablation in patients with primary and secondary hepatic malignancies. J Gastrointest Surg 2006; 10:960–73.

10. Abitabile P, Hartl U, Lange J, et al. Radiofrequency ablation permits an effective treatment for colorectal liver metastasis. Eur J Surg Oncol 2007;33:67–71.

11. van Duijnhoven FH, Jansen MC, Junggeburt JM, et al. Factors influencing the local failure rate of radiofrequency ablation of colorectal liver metastases. Ann Surg Oncol 2006;13:651–8.

12. Dodd GD 3rd, Frank MS, Aribandi M, et al. Radiofrequency thermal ablation: computer analysis of the size of the thermal injury created by overlapping ablations. AJR Am J Roentgenol 2001;177:777–82.

13. Jiang HC, Liu LX, Piao DX, et al. Clinical short-term results of radiofrequency ablation in liver cancers. World J Gastroenterol 2002;8:624–30.

14. Machi J, Uchida S, Sumida K, et al. Ultrasound-guided radiofrequency thermal ablation of liver tumors: percutaneous, laparoscopic, and open surgical approaches. J Gastrointest Surg 2001;5:477–89.

15. Joosten J, Jager G, Oyen W, et al. Cryosurgery and radiofrequency ablation for unresectable colorectal liver metastases. Eur J Surg Oncol 2005;31:1152–9.

16. Lu DS, Raman SS, Limanond P, et al. Influence of large peritumoral vessels on outcome of radiofrequency ablation of liver tumors. J Vasc Interv Radiol 2003;14: 1267–74.

17. Lu DS, Raman SS, Vodopich DJ, et al. Effect of vessel size on creation of hepatic radiofrequency lesions in pigs: assessment of the "heat sink" effect. AJR Am J Roentgenol 2002;178:47–51.

18. Okano K, Yamamoto J, Okabayashi T, et al. CT imaging of intrabiliary growth of colorectal liver metastases: a comparison of pathological findings of resected specimens. Br J Radiol 2002;75:497–501.

19. Parikh AA, Curley SA, Fornage BD, et al. Radiofrequency ablation of hepatic metastases. Semin Oncol 2002;29:168–82.

20. Goldberg SN, Grassi CJ, Cardella JF, et al. Image-guided tumor ablation: standardization of terminology and reporting criteria. Radiology 2005;235: 728–39.

21. Goldberg SN, Gazelle GS, Compton CC, et al. Treatment of intrahepatic malignancy with radiofrequency ablation: radiologic-pathologic correlation. Cancer 2000;88:2452–63.

22. Oyama Y, Nakamura K, Matsuoka T, et al. Radiofrequency ablated lesion in the normal porcine lung: long-term follow-up with MRI and pathology. Cardiovasc Intervent Radiol 2005;28:346–53.
23. Raman SS, Lu DS, Vodopich DJ, et al. Creation of radiofrequency lesions in a porcine model: correlation with sonography, CT, and histopathology. AJR Am J Roentgenol 2000;175:1253–8.
24. Park MH, Rhim H, Kim YS, et al. Spectrum of CT findings after radiofrequency ablation of hepatic tumors. Radiographics 2008;28:379–90 [discussion: 390–2].
25. Choi H, Loyer EM, DuBrow RA, et al. Radio-frequency ablation of liver tumors: assessment of therapeutic response and complications. Radiographics 2001; 21:S41–54.
26. Kim SK, Lim HK, Kim YH, et al. Hepatocellular carcinoma treated with radio-frequency ablation: spectrum of imaging findings. Radiographics 2003;23: 107–21.
27. Lim HK, Choi D, Lee WJ, et al. Hepatocellular carcinoma treated with percutaneous radio-frequency ablation: evaluation with follow-up multiphase helical CT. Radiology 2001;221:447–54.
28. Choi H, Evelyne M, Charnsangavej C. Radiographic imaging following radiofrequency ablation of liver tumors. In: Ellis LM, Curley SA, Tanabe KK, editors. Radiofrequency ablation for cancer: current indications, techniques, and outcomes. New York: Springer-Verlag; 2004. p. 253–67.
29. Goldberg SN, Gazelle GS, Solbiati L, et al. Ablation of liver tumors using percutaneous RF therapy. AJR Am J Roentgenol 1998;170:1023–8.
30. Sironi S, Livraghi T, Meloni F, et al. Small hepatocellular carcinoma treated with percutaneous RF ablation: MR imaging follow-up. AJR Am J Roentgenol 1999; 173:1225–9.
31. Dromain C, de Baere T, Elias D, et al. Hepatic tumors treated with percutaneous radio-frequency ablation: CT and MR imaging follow-up. Radiology 2002;223: 255–62.
32. Limanond P, Zimmerman P, Raman SS, et al. Interpretation of CT and MRI after radiofrequency ablation of hepatic malignancies. AJR Am J Roentgenol 2003; 181:1635–40.
33. McGhana JP, Dodd GD 3rd. Radiofrequency ablation of the liver: current status. AJR Am J Roentgenol 2001;176:3–16.
34. Goldberg SN, Gazelle GS, Mueller PR. Thermal ablation therapy for focal malignancy: a unified approach to underlying principles, techniques, and diagnostic imaging guidance. AJR Am J Roentgenol 2000;174:323–31.
35. Chopra S, Dodd GD 3rd, Chintapalli KN, et al. Tumor recurrence after radiofrequency thermal ablation of hepatic tumors: spectrum of findings on dual-phase contrast-enhanced CT. AJR Am J Roentgenol 2001;177:381–7.
36. Curley SA, Izzo F, Ellis LM, et al. Radiofrequency ablation of hepatocellular cancer in 110 patients with cirrhosis. Ann Surg 2000;232:381–91.
37. Akahane M, Koga H, Kato N, et al. Complications of percutaneous radiofrequency ablation for hepato-cellular carcinoma: imaging spectrum and management. Radiographics 2005;25(Suppl 1):S57–68.
38. Rhim H, Dodd GD 3rd, Chintapalli KN, et al. Radiofrequency thermal ablation of abdominal tumors: lessons learned from complications. Radiographics 2004;24: 41–52.
39. Rhim H, Lim HK, Kim YS, et al. Hemobilia after radiofrequency ablation of hepatocellular carcinoma. Abdom Imaging 2007;32:719–24.

40. Tamai F, Furuse J, Maru Y, et al. Intrahepatic pseudoaneurysm: a complication following radio-frequency ablation therapy for hepatocellular carcinoma. Eur J Radiol 2002;44:40–3.

41. Kim SK, Lim HK, Ryu JA, et al. Radiofrequency ablation of rabbit liver in vivo: effect of the Pringle maneuver on pathologic changes in liver surrounding the ablation zone. Korean J Radiol 2004;5:240–9.

42. Ng KK, Lam CM, Poon RT, et al. Delayed portal vein thrombosis after experimental radiofrequency ablation near the main portal vein. Br J Surg 2004;91:632–9.

43. Shen P, Fleming S, Westcott C, et al. Laparoscopic radiofrequency ablation of the liver in proximity to major vasculature: effect of the Pringle maneuver. J Surg Oncol 2003;83:36–41.

44. de Baere T, Risse O, Kuoch V, et al. Adverse events during radiofrequency treatment of 582 hepatic tumors. AJR Am J Roentgenol 2003;181:695–700.

45. Kim YS, Rhim H, Lim HK, et al. Hepatic infarction after radiofrequency ablation of hepatocellular carcinoma with an internally cooled electrode. J Vasc Interv Radiol 2007;18:1126–33.

46. Kim YS, Rhim H, Lim HK. Imaging after radiofrequency ablation of hepatic tumors. Semin Ultrasound CT MR 2009;30:49–66.

47. Livraghi T, Solbiati L, Meloni MF, et al. Treatment of focal liver tumors with percutaneous radio-frequency ablation: complications encountered in a multicenter study. Radiology 2003;226:441–51.

48. Chopra S, Dodd GD 3rd, Chanin MP, et al. Radiofrequency ablation of hepatic tumors adjacent to the gallbladder: feasibility and safety. AJR Am J Roentgenol 2003;180:697–701.

49. Choi D, Lim HK, Kim MJ, et al. Liver abscess after percutaneous radiofrequency ablation for hepatocellular carcinomas: frequency and risk factors. AJR Am J Roentgenol 2005;184:1860–7.

50. Mathieu D, Vasile N, Fagniez PL, et al. Dynamic CT features of hepatic abscesses. Radiology 1985;154:749–52.

51. Kim MD, Kim H, Kang SW, et al. Nontraumatic hepatic artery pseudoaneurysm associated with acute leukemia: a possible complication of pyogenic liver abscess. Abdom Imaging 2002;27:458–60.

52. Kim SH, Lim HK, Choi D, et al. Changes in bile ducts after radiofrequency ablation of hepatocellular carcinoma: frequency and clinical significance. AJR Am J Roentgenol 2004;183:1611–7.

53. Patterson EJ, Scudamore CH, Owen DA, et al. Radiofrequency ablation of porcine liver in vivo: effects of blood flow and treatment time on lesion size. Ann Surg 1998;227:559–65.

54. Hansen PD, Rogers S, Corless CL, et al. Radiofrequency ablation lesions in a pig liver model. J Surg Res 1999;87:114–21.

55. Krudy AG, Doppman JL, Bissonette MB, et al. Hemobilia: computed tomographic diagnosis. Radiology 1983;148:785–9.

56. Latteri F, Sandonato L, Di Marco V, et al. Seeding after radiofrequency ablation of hepatocellular carcinoma in patients with cirrhosis: a prospective study. Dig Liver Dis 2008;40:684–9.

57. Mulier S, Mulier P, Ni Y, et al. Complications of radiofrequency coagulation of liver tumours. Br J Surg 2002;89:1206–22.

58. Buscarini E, Buscarini L. Radiofrequency thermal ablation with expandable needle of focal liver malignancies: complication report. Eur Radiol 2004;14:31–7.

59. Jaskolka JD, Asch MR, Kachura JR, et al. Needle tract seeding after radiofrequency ablation of hepatic tumors. J Vasc Interv Radiol 2005;16:485–91.

Ablative Therapies of the Breast

Ranjna Sharma, MD[a],*, Jamie L. Wagner, DO[b],
Rosa F. Hwang, MD[b]

KEYWORDS

- Breast cancer • Ablation • Radiofrequency ablation
- Cryoablation

Over the past 5 decades, the treatment of breast cancer has evolved from highly invasive radical mastectomies to breast-conserving therapy that allows women to avoid severe disfigurement and related morbidity while providing equivalent survival benefit.[1–3] More recently, the approach for nodal staging has also become less invasive with the adoption of sentinel lymph node biopsy as the current standard of care for patients with early-stage breast cancer.[4–6]

Continuing with this trend toward minimally invasive therapy, various ablative techniques have been studied for the treatment of breast cancer. Both thermal and cold techniques have been evaluated as potential treatment modalities. Radiofrequency ablation, interstitial laser therapy, high-intensity focused ultrasonography, and focused microwave ablation result in tumor destruction from significant heating of the tissue. Cryoablation is the technique that causes tumor destruction through extreme cooling of the tissue. This article gives an overview of the technical aspects of each procedure, along with the advantages, disadvantages, and evidence of their efficacy.

RADIOFREQUENCY ABLATION
Technical Aspects of Radiofrequency Ablation

Radiofrequency ablation (RFA) has been used for the treatment of liver metastases, primary hepatocellular carcinoma, pulmonary neoplasia, and renal cell carcinoma.[7] RFA is performed by placing electrode tips within the lesion, creating a high-frequency alternating current into the surrounding tissue. The ions in the tissue attempt to follow the changing direction, causing ion agitation and thus frictional heating of the tissue.

The authors did not receive any financial support toward writing this article.
The authors have no financial disclosures or conflicts of interest.
[a] Breast Care Center, Department of Surgery, Beth Israel Deaconess Medical Center, Harvard Medical School, Shapiro 5, 330 Brookline Avenue, Boston, MA 02215, USA
[b] Department of Surgical Oncology, University of Texas MD Anderson Cancer Center, 1400 Holcombe Boulevard, Unit 444, Houston, TX 77030, USA
* Corresponding author.
E-mail address: rsharma1@bidmc.harvard.edu

Surg Oncol Clin N Am 20 (2011) 317–339
doi:10.1016/j.soc.2010.11.003
1055-3207/11/$ – see front matter © 2011 Elsevier Inc. All rights reserved.

This process results in destruction of the tissue through thermal coagulation and protein denaturation.[8–10] Thermal injury begins at 40°C, with the exposure time necessary for cell death decreasing exponentially at 42.5°C. Temperatures generated by the electrode must be much greater than 50°C to achieve cell death, as most human tumors require temperatures greater than 45°C to 50°C.[8] The multipronged RFA probe is most commonly placed under sonographic guidance and the procedure performed during real-time sonographic monitoring. Treatment is completed once the tumor has been heated to a specific temperature or once tissue impedance has reached a level at which no further heating can occur.[8,11,12]

Treatment of Invasive Breast Cancer with Radiofrequency Ablation

RFA has been described for the treatment of invasive breast carcinoma.[13–17] Jeffrey and colleagues[13] reported a small series of 5 women with tumor sizes ranging from 4 to 7 cm measured by clinical examination or mammography at the time of the procedure, who were treated with RFA at a single site within the tumor under ultrasound guidance. Following RFA, 4 patients underwent modified radical mastectomy and 1 underwent breast-conserving surgery. Complete loss of cell viability, as determined by NADH-diaphorase staining, was observed in the tumors of 4 patients, while a single small area (<1 mm) of cell viability was identified in one patient's tumor. Hematoxylin and eosin (H&E) staining revealed 2 patients with necrosis of all cells and 3 patients with normal-appearing cells interspersed between necrotic cells. Although only a small number of patients were included, the results of this study were encouraging to further evaluate RFA in a larger group of patients.

The first prospective clinical protocol to evaluate RFA for invasive breast cancer was reported by Fornage and colleagues[14] at the University of Texas MD Anderson Cancer Center. Twenty patients with 21 tumors that were well visualized on sonography were included, and all patients had tumors measuring 2 cm or less in greatest diameter, with 1 cm between the tumor and skin and tumor and chest wall. The RFA procedure was performed percutaneously under ultrasound guidance in the operating room immediately before the scheduled surgical procedure. Eleven patients underwent partial mastectomy and 9 underwent total mastectomy. Sentinel lymph node mapping was performed prior to the RFA procedure. Ultrasound changes as a result of thermal injury were monitored at random intervals throughout the RFA procedure. Only a single RFA ablation session was needed in all but one tumor. No skin or chest wall complications were identified intraoperative or postoperatively. On histologic examination of the surgical specimen, all tumors were found to have cellular damage and thermal effect (as observed on H&E staining) as well as complete ablation (determined by NADH-diaphorase staining). The studies by Fornage and colleagues and others[15–17] that evaluate RFA within a short time period before the excision of the primary tumor are all limited because cell death can be delayed for 48 hours following ablation. In addition, evaluation of complications is limited by excision of the lesion and overlying skin that may have been affected.

To assess the delayed effects of RFA, Manenti and colleagues[18] performed RFA followed by surgical resection 1 month later. This study enrolled 34 postmenopausal women with biopsy-proven, unifocal, invasive ductal carcinoma 2 cm or less in size, visible on both ultrasonography and magnetic resonance imaging (MRI) that was at least 1 cm from the skin and chest wall on sonography. Sentinel lymph node biopsy was performed at the time of the RFA procedure. MRI was performed 1 week and 4 weeks following RFA to determine the accuracy of MRI in predicting the efficacy of RFA. Definitive surgical intervention with lumpectomy was performed at 4 weeks post-RFA in all patients. Seven patients with positive sentinel nodes underwent axillary lymph node dissection. Patients also received breast irradiation or adjuvant systemic therapy according to St Gallen oncologic criteria, and hormonal therapy was given in accordance with the biopsy hormonal receptor status. H&E staining of surgical specimens showed a spectrum of changes, from partial (6% [2/34] of patients) to complete changes (94% [32/34] of patients). In addition, NADH-diaphorase revealed no viable cells in 97% (33/34) of the tumors. One week after ablation, MRI showed no residual suspicious enhancement in 31 of 34 lesions, although residual enhancement was present in the remaining 3 lesions. The correlation between MRI findings and pathology of the specimens was not described except in one patient in whom NADH-diaphorase staining confirmed residual cancer at the site of enhancement on MRI. Cosmesis was rated as excellent in 82% (28/34) of patients, good in 15% (5/34), and poor in 3% (1/34). Suboptimal cosmetic outcomes were attributed to the formation of a mass as a result of thermocoagulation and hyperpigmentation from superficial skin burn.[18]

Finally, studies have been performed in which the primary tumor was not excised following RFA, with the objective of assessing recurrence.[19–22] Oura and colleagues[20] evaluated 52 patients with small (2 cm) localized breast cancers, confirmed on mammography, sonography, and MRI, who underwent RFA. Sentinel lymph node dissection was performed before the RFA procedure. The RFA needle was inserted from the areola into the tumor under ultrasound guidance. Cytologic evaluation performed 3 to 4 weeks post-RFA (presumably by percutaneous biopsy) revealed degenerative cancer cells in 30 patients and no cancer cells and/or degenerative materials in 22 patients. MRI performed 1 to 3 months after RFA revealed no evidence of residual tumor in the ablation zone. Ultrasonography showed residual tumor in 30 of the 52 patients, although no vascular flow was seen in any of the cases. With a mean follow-up of 15 months (range, 6–30 months), no patients had developed in-breast recurrence, locoregional recurrence (LRR), or distant recurrence. Cosmesis was determined to be excellent or good in 43 and 6 patients (83% and 11%), and fair in 3 patients (6%). One patient did experience a skin burn, identified shortly after biopsy. Similarly, in a pilot study of 29 patients (30 breasts) by Yamamoto and colleagues,[22] no hypervascularity of the tumor in the ablated zone was found in any patient on post-RFA MRI. However, H&E staining of post-RFA tumor specimens obtained by vacuum-assisted biopsy was performed in 3 of the 29 breasts, revealing remarkable degenerative changes. The remaining tumors were diagnosed as containing viable tumor tissue. NADH-diaphorase staining showed no viable tumor tissue in 24 of the 26 patients in whom it was performed. Adverse events occurred in 4 out of 29 patients in this study. Fibrotic tissue was present in the tumors of all patients, confirming the absence of viable malignant cells in the samples analyzed.

Most studies using RFA have focused on using the minimally invasive approach for the treatment of invasive breast carcinoma. However, a novel role of RFA as an adjunct to surgical excision (eRFA) has been explored[23] in an attempt to decrease the rate of reexcision and improve locoregional recurrence. In a pilot study, RFA was performed on an ex vivo lumpectomy specimen in 19 patients. Proliferation cell nuclear antigen (PCNA) staining confirmed 100% nonviable tissue within the ablation zones. In a subsequent group of 41 patients with T1 and T2 tumors (mean tumor size 1.6 cm), standard lumpectomy was followed immediately by eRFA. On final pathology, 10 patients had close margins (8 with 1 mm, 1 with 2 mm margin, 1 with focally positive margin) and none of these patients underwent re-resection. Seventeen patients received post-eRFA breast irradiation (41%). Two patients developed recurrent cancer in the same breast. One patient developed a new invasive lobular carcinoma 1 year following excision and RFA of ductal carcinoma in situ (DCIS). The recurrent tumor was located 8 cm from the primary tumor site. The second patient developed a new grade II invasive carcinoma following treatment of a grade III primary tumor 2.3 years after treatment, and the recurrent lesion was located 5 cm from the primary tumor site. Both patients were successfully treated with salvage mastectomy.[23]

Conclusion

Although initial studies in the use of RFA for the treatment of early-stage breast cancer appear hopeful, there are several issues that need consideration before the technique can be widely adopted. The availability of pre-RFA tissue to evaluate estrogen, progesterone, and HER 2/neu status is imperative because loss of hormonal and HER 2/neu expression can occur with RFA treatment. In addition, RFA may potentially alter the lymphatic drainage pattern of the breast tumor. Thus, the timing of sentinel lymph node biopsy in conjunction with ablative techniques is controversial.[14,18,22] To date, there have been no prospective trials to evaluate the influence of the RFA procedure on sentinel lymph node biopsy. To accurately assess the efficacy of RFA for invasive breast cancer, the technique must be evaluated in a prospective fashion with concomitant evaluation of resected surgical specimens. Resection should be performed at least 48 hours after RFA to allow for delayed histologic changes, and NADH-diaphorase staining may also be helpful in assessing cell viability. Thus far, RFA with subsequent surgical excision has only been evaluated prospectively in a relatively small number of patients. Thus, further evaluation in a larger number of patients with longer follow-up is needed to determine its role in the treatment of invasive breast cancer.

CRYOTHERAPY

Cryoablation is an ablative therapy that is receiving increasing attention and is being used with increased frequency, due to improvements and advances in imaging and cold technology. It has already been studied in tumors of the liver, prostate, and kidney.[24–31] Cryoablation is another example of a minimally invasive approach under investigation to treat breast tumors, both benign and malignant.

Technical Aspects of Cryoablation

The technique of cryoablation uses cold technology to destroy a breast tumor in situ via localized freezing. After infiltration of local anesthetic, a small incision a few millimeters in size is created for percutaneous cryoprobe placement (**Fig. 1**). The probe is inserted into the tumor via image guidance (usually ultrasound; however, computed tomography and MRI have also been reported)[29,30,32–35] through a trocar (**Fig. 2**). Nitrogen or argon gas (cryogen) flow is initiated into the probe tip via a computer modulated regulator. The gas undergoes a constant enthalpy expansion process, allowing a rapid local freezing reaction to occur. Then a second gas, such as helium, which warms when it expands, is released through the probe to arrest the freezing process and allow thawing to actively occur.[32,33,36,37] The thawing process can also occur passively by discontinuing the flow of argon and allowing the probe to warm.[32,33,38,39] This cycle is repeated and results in tissue necrosis. A complete treatment consists of at least 2 freeze-thaw cycles, with cycle length in minutes based on tumor diameter.[32,33,35,36,38,40] Tissues exposed to at least 2 consecutive freeze-thaw cycles at temperatures of $-40°C$ or lower will allow consistent and symmetric ablation to occur.[29,36,39,40] An ice ball is created, which can be easily visualized on intraprocedural ultrasonography by visualizing the hyperechoic rim that forms between frozen and unfrozen tissue (**Fig. 3**).[39,40] The ice ball that forms creates a uniform ablation zone, providing an even field of distribution for the cryotherapy process, resulting

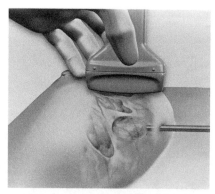

Fig. 1. Cryoprobe placement into tumor under ultrasound guidance. (*Reprinted from* Kaufman CS, Littrup PJ, Freman-Gibb LA, et al. Office-based cryoablation of breast fibroadenomas: 12-month follow-up. J Am Coll Surg 2004;198:915; Copyright 2004, with permission from Elsevier.)

in homogeneous tissue necrosis.[36,40,41] However, there are reports that there is inconsistent cell death at the periphery of the ice ball resulting from differences in cellular exposure to the freezing temperatures of the cryoablation process, thus supporting the need for a double freeze-thaw cycle.[27,40] The frozen tissue that has been created remains in situ and is reabsorbed by the body over time.[39] Continuous ultrasound monitoring is used to monitor the extent of freezing based on the size of the forming ice ball.[33] Saline can be injected between the tumor and overlying skin if there is a distance of less than 5 mm from the ice ball to the skin surface to prevent thermal injury to the skin from occurring (**Fig. 4**). In this manner, superficial tumors may be

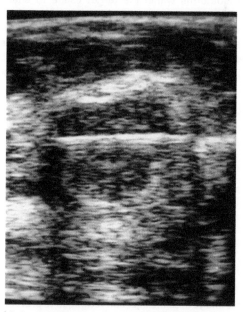

Fig. 2. Ultrasonographic image of cryoprobe through tumor. (*Reprinted from* Kaufman CS, Bachman B, Littrup PJ, et al. Cryoablation treatment of benign breast lesions with 12-month follow-up. Am J Surg 2004;188:341; Copyright 2004, with permission from Elsevier.)

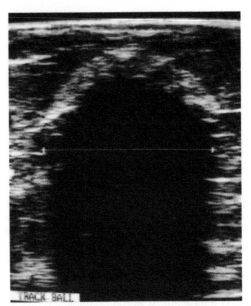

Fig. 3. Ultrasonographic image of ice ball formation during cryoablation. (*Reprinted from* Kaufman CS, Bachman B, Littrup PJ, et al. Cryoablation treatment of benign breast lesions with 12-month follow-up. Am J Surg 2004;188:346; Copyright 2004, with permission from Elsevier.)

treated.[32,33,35,36] In patients who have larger tumors, multiple cryoprobes may be used to generate multiple isotherms within the target tissue to ensure complete tumor ablation.[29,32,33,38–40] Of note, a core-needle biopsy needs to be performed prior to tumor ablation so that adequate tissue can be obtained both for a histopathologic diagnosis and for the determination of tumor receptor (ER, PR, Her2neu) status.

Tumor cells are destroyed in 2 ways, via direct cell injury and via indirect vasculature injury. In direct cell injury intracellular ice formation occurs, causing a shearing and

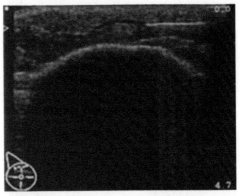

Fig. 4. Ultrasonographic image of saline injection technique to prevent overlying skin injury. (*Reprinted from* Whitworth PW, Rewcastle JC. Cryoablation and cryolocalization in the management of breast disease. J Surg Oncol 2005;90:3; Copyright 2005, with permission from John Wiley & Sons Inc.)

rupture of membranes, which is an irreversible event. Extracellular ice formation occurs, creating a hypertonic environment and causing water to flow out of cells due to osmosis. This process, referred to as "solution effect injury," causes cellular dehydration and damage. When thawing occurs, water flows back into the cell, increasing the intracellular volume and causing lysis to occur (**Fig. 5**).[27,28,32,33,35,36,39,40,42,43] Vascular injury occurs when the freezing process causes vasoconstriction. The vasoconstrictive process causes ischemia to occur, which results in damage to the microvascular endothelium. Platelet aggregation occurs, resulting in thrombosis and vascular stasis. This loss of circulation causes cellular anoxia and death[27,28,35,36,40,44] as well as the production of free radicals.[27,35]

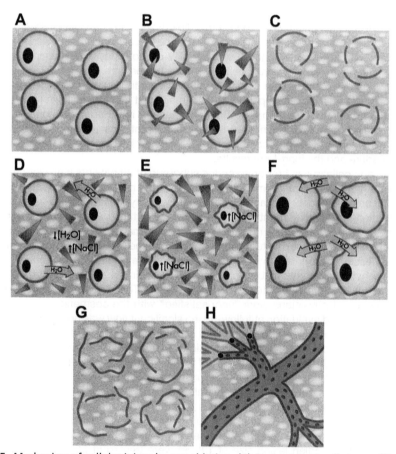

Fig. 5. Mechanism of cellular injury by cryoablation. (*A*) Pretreatment cells in equilibrium. (*B*) Intracellular ice formation. (*C*) Extreme cooling causes shearing of cell membranes. (*D*) Extracellular ice formation leads to hypertonic extracellular space and compensatory exit of water from cells; (*E*) this creates a hypertonic intracellular environment. (*F*) Thawing causes rush of water back into cells. (*G*) Resultant rupturing of cell membranes and cell lysis. (*H*) In addition, there is capillary endothelial damage that creates delayed thrombosis and local hypoxia (at 3–5 days). (*Reprinted from* Kaufman CS, Littrup PJ, Freman-Gibb LA, et al. Office-based cryoablation of breast fibroadenomas: 12-month follow-up. J Am Coll Surg 2004;198:916; Copyright 2004, with permission from Elsevier.)

Cryoablation as Therapy for Benign Breast Tumors

Because benign breast tumors are very common and can cause a significant amount of anxiety, fear, discomfort, need for ongoing surveillance, and impaired visualization on follow-up imaging due to mass effect from the tumor, definitive treatment in the form of cryoablation is a viable option for patients who do not desire surgery or are not candidates for general anesthesia or surgical resection.[44] Several investigators have evaluated the efficacy of cryoablation for benign breast tumors. Kaufman and colleagues[44] reported on a series of 57 patients with fibroadenomas of the breast treated in a prospective nonrandomized multicenter trial who received cryoablation as their primary therapy. The mean maximum tumor diameter was 2.1 cm. After histopathologic confirmation of a fibroadenoma by core biopsy, patients underwent cryotherapy using 2 freeze-thaw cycles, with freezing occurring at −40°C. Following cryoablation, patients were followed with clinical examination, ultrasonography, core-needle biopsy, and patient satisfaction surveys. Long-term follow-up results for 29 patients were available, with an average follow-up time of 2.6 years. The efficacy analysis showed a continuous decrease in tumor palpability and visibility on both physical examination and imaging, respectively, as tissue debris resorbed over time. Only 16% of lesions remained palpable at the time of last follow-up. A median volume reduction of 99% of the original tumor occurred per ultrasound imaging at the time of last follow-up. No major complications were reported; although 3 patients reported minor complications of tenderness (2) and cyclic pain (1). Ninety-seven percent of patients reported satisfaction with the results of the procedure, and 100% of physicians reported satisfaction with the procedure and the long-term results.

Littrup and colleagues[32] reported on the subgroup of 29 patients who were treated at a single institution from the multicenter trial reported by Kaufman and colleagues[44] These 29 patients had 42 fibroadenomas treated with cryotherapy. Thirty-seven of the 42 fibroadenomas had 12 months of follow-up. In 33 of these 37 patients, their fibroadenoma had either completely resolved or was much smaller on physical examination. None of these patients exhibited skin changes over the treated area or evidence of skin depression secondary to volume reduction at the treated site. Although there was initial hypopigmentation at the probe insertion site in 3 patients, this had resolved at 12-month follow-up; one patient developed a keloid. The investigators reported that both patient and physicians were "very satisfied" with the cosmetic outcomes. On Doppler ultrasound evaluation at follow-up, no significant flow was noted in the treated area, whereas there was normalized flow in the adjacent untreated tissue. By 12 months, continued shrinkage and resorption rendered 5 of the fibroadenomas no longer visible by ultrasound imaging. All of the patients were offered the opportunity to undergo surgical resection if they were unsatisfied with the results of the cryoablation; only 2 patients chose to have a formal resection.[32]

Nurko and colleagues[41] reported results from the prospective Fibroadenoma Cryoablation Treatment Registry, which includes patients with breast fibroadenomas treated with cryotherapy in a community setting. Four hundred and forty-four fibroadenomas with a median lesion size of 1.8 cm were treated at 55 different practice sites. After placement of the cryoprobe through the long axis of the fibroadenoma, 2 freeze-thaw cycles at probe temperatures of −160°C were used for treatment. Patients were followed at 12 months with clinical examination and ultrasound imaging. Thirty-five percent of the tumors that were initially palpable were palpable at 12 months for the 82 patients for whom this information was available. Ultrasound imaging showed the reabsorbing lesion in 29% of the 71 patients for whom this information was available. Patient satisfaction at 12 months was high (88%) in 84 patients.

In contrast to surgical excision, cryoablation of fibroadenomas results in decreased morbidity from ductal damage and incisional pain, decreased patient distress, and improved cosmesis.[36] As many physicians are reluctant to allow a lump to remain in situ in a woman who may not be motivated toward appropriate follow-up, cryoablation represents an effective minimally invasive alternative to surgical excision in these patients who have a biopsy-proven benign process.[36,41]

Cryoablation of Invasive Breast Carcinoma

More recently, the role of cryoablation in the treatment of malignant breast tumors has been evaluated, primarily in early-stage cancers. Pfleiderer and colleagues[38] treated 15 patients with 16 early-stage breast cancers (9–40 mm diameter) with cryoablation. Each patient underwent ultrasound-guided cryotherapy consisting of 2 freeze-thaw cycles under local anesthesia, followed by surgical resection 5 days after the cryoablation procedure. No major complications were reported. In patients whose tumor size was 1.5 cm or less, there was no residual invasive carcinoma in the pathologic specimens. In patients whose tumors were larger than 1.5 cm there was incomplete tumor destruction, with remnants of invasive carcinoma present in the histopathologic specimens. The investigators recommended the use of multiple cryoprobes to effectively treat larger lesions. In a follow-up study, Pfleiderer and colleagues[43] prospectively evaluated 30 patients with biopsy-proven breast carcinoma (invasive and in situ) 15 mm or less in size who underwent cryoablation. Twenty-nine patients successfully underwent ultrasound-guided cryotherapy with 2 freeze-thaw cycles, with a median minimum temperature of −146°C. No major complications were reported. All patients underwent surgical resection within 6 weeks. No invasive tumor cells were identified in any of the patients, whereas DCIS was identified outside of the ablation zone in 5 patients, raising the question of the accuracy of pretreatment imaging in defining the extent of disease.

Sabel and colleagues[33] performed a multi-institutional pilot study to assess safety and feasibility of cryotherapy in the treatment of early breast cancer. Twenty-nine patients with T1 tumors were enrolled in the study; 27 patients successfully underwent cryoablation with a double freeze-thaw cycle with a probe temperature of −160°C. Most patients (25/27) had the procedure performed under local anesthesia. All patients then had a formal oncologic surgical resection 7 to 30 days after the cryotherapy. Twenty-five of these 27 patients underwent a sentinel lymph node biopsy at the time of the surgical resection, with 4 patients having carcinoma identified in the sentinel node. There were no major complications. Minor complications that were reported include tenderness, edema, and ecchymosis. Cryotherapy successfully ablated 100% of carcinoma cells in tumors that were less than 1.0 cm in diameter. In patients who had tumors that were between 1.0 and 1.5 cm, cryoablation achieved 100% success only if the tumor did not contain a significant amount of DCIS. In patients who had DCIS present without calcifications, cryotherapy was not reliable. The investigators showed that cryoablation was safe and well tolerated in an office-based setting, with reliable results of complete eradication of all carcinoma cells in patients with ductal or medullary tumors less than 1.5 cm in size who did not have extensive intraductal component (EIC). Thus, the success of the procedure was based on the size of the cancer and the histology of the tumor. Sabel and colleagues also showed that sentinel lymph node biopsy could be performed after cryotherapy, although the false-negative rate was not specifically determined in this study. As breast cancers are detected at much earlier stages nowadays because of the increased screening and improved imaging techniques, having an alternative to surgical resection that produces less pain, improved cosmesis, and decreased costs is advantageous.[33,38,43]

The studies by Pfleiderer and colleagues[38,43] and Sabel and colleagues[33] show that cryoablation can be used for definitive destruction of breast carcinoma in select patients. Tumor size and histology are important criteria in defining the appropriate patient population. Tumors must be unifocal and visible on preoperative imaging. Sentinel lymph node biopsy is feasible after cryoablation has been performed,[33] although the issue of accuracy in this setting still needs to be evaluated.

Additional Roles for Cryoablation in the Treatment of Breast Cancer

Cryoablation can also be used for tumor localization prior to lumpectomy for nonpalpable lesions, similar to the needle-wire localization technique. To achieve this localization, a cryoprobe is used to enclose a nonpalpable or barely palpable tumor (with surrounding tissue margin) in a rim of ice under ultrasound guidance immediately before a formal breast-conserving surgical resection, creating a template for the resective procedure.[36,37,45,46] This technique eliminates the need for an additional procedure outside the operating room, as is the case with needle-wire localization, and also minimizes the possibility of displacement of the localization device during patient transfer.[37,45] In addition, the frozen tissue is more firm and easier to manipulate during surgical resection.[37,45] Also, this procedure may potentially decrease local recurrence, likely by encapsulating the tumor and thus preventing the spillage of tumor cells during surgical resection.[33,39,46,47] Of note, a core-needle biopsy would also need to be performed before surgical excision via the cryo-assisted lumpectomy technique, to ensure an accurate histopathologic diagnosis and receptor status identification because of the occurrence of freezing artifact after cryotherapy.[37]

In addition, cryotherapy can be used for local-regional palliation of locally advanced breast cancer and Stage 4 disease.[47,48] Tanaka[48] treated 49 patients who had locally advanced, metastatic, or recurrent breast cancer with cryotherapy, which resulted in an improvement of symptoms. Specifically, the patients had less pain, control of hemorrhage, and tumor volume reduction, with a 5-year survival rate of 44%. Suzuki[47] reviewed 8 patients who had locally advanced breast cancer with distant metastasis in whom the primary tumor was treated with cryotherapy. Cryoablation reportedly palliated symptoms of the primary breast tumor and palliated distant disease symptoms consisting of dyspnea due to a pleural effusion in one patient and lower extremity paralysis and incontinence due to vertebral metastases in another patient.

Several preclinical studies suggest that cryoablation may decrease local recurrence and distant metastases. In a murine model of breast cancer, cryoablation caused a tumor-specific immunologic response with a release of cytokines interleukin-12 and interferon-γ, and increased natural killer cell activity.[42,43,47] This immune response may be able to prevent local recurrence and distant metastases.[33,42,47] Sabel and colleagues[42] have also recently reported a decrease in pulmonary metastases and an increase in survival in a murine model after cryoablation with a high freeze rate. Thus, a theoretical systemic antitumor response is created. In addition, cryoablated tissue has a surrounding hypervascular rim, which may have implications for delivery of chemotherapy or increased sensitization to radiation therapy.[32,40]

Advantages of cryoablation include patient comfort, as the ice ball that is produced has an analgesic effect, minimizing the patient's intraprocedural and postprocedural discomfort.[28,32,33,36–38,41] There is improved cosmesis when compared with lumpectomy (without tissue rearrangement), as there is no volume reduction, retraction, or concavity within the breast tissue nor is there a large surgical scar (**Fig. 6**).[27,32,37,39] Also, the shape of the breast is maintained because the collagenous framework is preserved during the cryotherapy process.[32] There is also increased convenience when compared with surgical procedures, as cryoablation can be performed in an

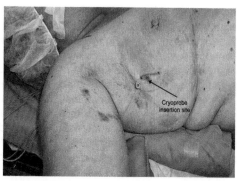

Fig. 6. Minimally invasive cryoablative therapy provides optimal cosmetic result.

outpatient setting without the use of general anesthesia, also decreasing overall costs.[28,32,33,35,37,38,41,44] The procedure is well tolerated, and patients report a high degree of satisfaction with the treatment and the cosmetic results.[32,36,41,44]

Disadvantages of cryoablative therapy center on the fact that certain staging information may be lost, due to a complete pathologic specimen not being produced; specifically, tumor size and margin status. Accurately defining tumor margins in relationship to the treatment field during and after the procedure is important.[32,33] If this information is lacking, recommendations for adjuvant therapies may be altered or unclear. There is concern that the accuracy and ability to perform sentinel lymph node biopsy may be lost because of disrupted lymphatics if a sentinel lymph node biopsy is not performed before cryoablation, due to disruption of lymphatic channels that may occur with cryotherapy. However, Sabel and colleagues[33] have reported that it is feasible to perform sentinel lymph node biopsy after a cryoablation. Also, it is also important to perform a core biopsy before cryoablation, ensuring enough tissue is obtained for an accurate diagnosis and tumor receptor status. Another disadvantage of cryoablation is that the ice ball that is created can remain for approximately 1 month after the procedure before it is resorbed by the body, interfering with physical examination or obscuring postprocedure imaging. The larger the tumor and subsequently formed ice ball, the longer it takes for resorption to occur.[30,41] Also, current imaging modalities are limited in their ability to detect in situ carcinoma. Thus, if preablation imaging does not accurately define the extent of disease, cryotherapy may not destroy all in situ and invasive cancer.[33]

Complications of the procedure include ecchymosis and hematoma formation. Thermal injury to the overlying skin in the form of ulceration or necrosis may also occur. As previously mentioned, this skin injury can be minimized with the injection of saline into the tissue between the tumor and the overlying skin. Minor complications include pain and tenderness at the site of the procedure. Postprocedural edema has also been reported.[33,44]

Postprocedural monitoring can be performed with a variety of imaging modalities, including mammography, ultrasonography, or MRI. These imaging modalities allow visualization of the ice ball that has been created as a result of the ablative procedure.[32] Ultrasound imaging shows the ablated tissue becoming more hypoechoic over time, as it involutes, resorbs, and reorganizes.[32,41] Following treatment, Littrup and colleagues[32] reported that color Doppler evaluation showed no significant flow in the cryoablation zone. Tissue sampling can also be performed to ensure that no cancer cells remain within a specimen, if the procedure is being performed in patients with breast carcinoma.

The American College of Surgeons Oncology Group is currently enrolling patients in a prospective, multi-institutional, phase 2 trial, ACOSOG-Z1072, cosponsored by the National Cancer Institute, that is investigating the rate of complete tumor destruction in patients with T1 unifocal invasive ductal carcinoma treated with cryotherapy. Secondary end points include the evaluation of the negative predictive value of MRI to detect residual disease, adverse events assessment, pain assessment, and evaluation of technical variables affecting the cryoablation procedure. Patients must undergo a core-needle biopsy for diagnosis and to determine receptor status prior to cryoablation. Cryoablation of the breast cancer will be followed by surgical resection and lymph node evaluation within 28 days (**Fig. 7**). Imaging follow-up will occur with MRI. To be eligible for this study, patients may not have received neoadjuvant chemotherapy.[49,50]

In conclusion, cryoablation may represent an alternative to surgical resection for breast tumors. It is an office-based procedure that causes minimal patient discomfort with improved cosmetic outcomes, and has potentially reduced costs. Cryotherapy has been shown to be a safe and feasible treatment for breast fibroadenomas. Current ongoing prospective multicenter trials, such as ACOSOG Z1072, will evaluate its efficacy in the treatment of breast carcinoma and determine whether a secondary immunologic response occurs with cryoablation that may alter the rate of local-regional recurrence and distant metastases. Long-term results from prospective trials will be necessary before cryoablation can replace breast conservation therapy in selected patients with early breast cancer.

OTHER ABLATIVE THERAPIES

Other ablative therapies used to treat breast tumors include interstitial laser therapy, high-intensity focused ultrasonography, and focused microwave therapy. These therapies rely on hyperthermia to destroy tumor cells where the amount of thermal injury is affected by the absolute temperature and exposure time. As a tissue's temperature increases, the time needed for cell death decreases.[36] These therapies cause the melting and fusion of cellular membranes and protein denaturation, which causes irreversible cell death.[42] Breast tissue is composed of fat cells and stromal elements, which have different heat capacities and thermal impedance, thus conducting heat at different rates.[36,44] Thus, a potential limitation to any hyperthermic ablative process is a less uniform necrosis that is produced, when compared with cold ablative therapy, due to the physical properties of breast tissue.[44] In addition, the hyperthermic ablation

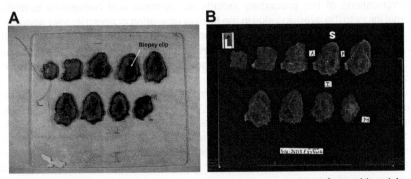

Fig. 7. (*A*) Pathologic sectioning of a surgical resection specimen of cryoablated breast tissue. (*B*) Radiographic imaging of a surgical resection specimen of cryoablated tissue, where circular outlines mark the site of tumor.

process does produce pain, usually necessitating the use of conscious sedation or general anesthesia during the procedure, and postoperative analgesia.[36] Also, there is the concern of thermal injury to the overlying skin, causing difficulty in treating superficial tumors. It has been recommended that a distance of 1 cm between the tumor and the skin surface be observed to avoid burns.[33] As with the other ablative therapies already reviewed, the approaches that are reviewed in this section may be preferable to surgical excision with regard to decreased costs, less morbidity, and improved cosmesis.

Interstitial Laser Therapy

Interstitial laser therapy is a hyperthermic percutaneous minimally invasive treatment that has been studied for early breast cancers. The procedure produces a refraction of laser light at the targeted tissue, where near-infrared photons are absorbed. This phenomenon produces heat, which causes coagulation necrosis and protein denaturation, leading to irreversible tissue destruction.[51–53] Initially, the temperature within the tissue increases uniformly. Then a temperature gradient develops between the center of the tumor and its periphery, not exceeding the set temperature maximum so as to prevent tissue carbonization and vaporization from occurring.[54] This process causes a direct cytotoxic effect on cancer cells and damages the endothelial cells of the tumor's microvasculature.[55]

Dowlatshahi and colleagues[51,56] have described the procedure of stereotactically guided interstitial laser therapy for the treatment of early breast cancer. Patients initially underwent core-needle biopsy for diagnosis and to determine hormone receptor status. At the start of the procedure patients were placed supine on a stereotactic table, immobilizing the breast to be treated. The volume of the treatment field was calculated by measuring the largest diameter of the lesion with a 0.5-cm rim of tissue surrounding it, using the formula for volume of a sphere ($V = 4/3\Pi\ r^3$). This calculated volume determined the amount of laser energy required to completely ablate the tumor, with the investigators' experimental data showing that 1400 J of energy was needed to eradicate 1 mL of breast tissue. Under intravenous sedation and local anesthesia, a laser probe was percutaneously inserted into the center of the tumor under mammographic guidance. Thermal sensors attached to the laser probe were used to measure the temperature in the central region of the tumor and the periphery of the treatment sphere (**Fig. 8**). Stereotactic images were obtained to confirm the position of both probes. A fluid pump was attached to the laser probe to deliver a normal saline infusion to the breast tissue and to serve as a coolant during the ablative procedure, preventing the central temperature from exceeding 100°C. Laser energy was delivered until the peripheral temperature reached 60°C or the precalculated amount of energy had been administered.[51,56]

Using this technique,[51] 36 patients with invasive (34) or in situ (2) breast carcinoma (<2 cm) were treated. The patients were treated with a mean energy level of 5650 J, achieving a temperature range between 80°C and 100°C for the central sensor and 60°C for the peripheral sensor. Lumpectomy was performed within 1 to 8 weeks after laser thermotherapy. Histopathologic analysis of the surgical specimens showed complete tumor necrosis in 24 (67%) patients, which corresponded to the tumors treated with 2500 J/mL. The remaining 12 patients showed viable tumor cells at the periphery of the tumor, likely due to inadequate energy delivery, laser probe displacement or malfunction, suboptimal visualization of the tumor mass, or large tumor size. Although 2 patients experienced minor skin burns at the site of laser probe entry and some patients complained of mild pain during the procedure, no major complications were reported.[51] In a subsequent study, the investigators addressed the issue of

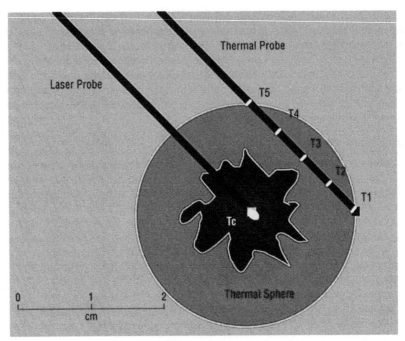

Fig. 8. Sketch of a breast cancer with associated laser and thermal probes during interstitial laser therapy. The laser probe with an attached thermal sensor (Tc) records the central temperature. The multisensor (T1–T5) thermal probe records the temperature of concentric zones around the tumor. (*Reprinted from* Dowlatshahi K, Fan M, Gould VE, et al. Stereotactically guided laser therapy for occult breast tumors. Arch Surg 2000;135:1347; Copyright 2000, American Medical Association; with permission.)

suboptimal visualization of the tissue mass by inserting metallic clips around the tumor before initiation of the ablative procedure.[56]

In a study from the Netherlands, van Esser and colleagues[53] examined laser ablation therapy in 14 patients with biopsy-proven breast cancer whose tumors were clinically 2.0 cm or less in size. Each tumor was treated with 7 W of energy, for a mean treatment time of 21 minutes. Complications from the procedure included 1 patient with a skin burn and 1 patient with a pneumothorax that was treated conservatively. In 7 of the 14 (50%) patients, the carcinoma was completely ablated on histopathologic evaluation. Of note, on pathologic evaluation 6 tumors were larger than 2.0 cm. Among this group of 6 patients, only 1 patient had complete tumor destruction. The investigators concluded that interstitial laser thermotherapy was feasible in the treatment of invasive ductal breast cancers 2.0 cm or less in size, without EIC. Van Esser and colleagues also cited the need for more accurate preprocedural imaging to define tumor size, listing lobular histology, presence of EIC, and angioinvasion as reasons for size discrepancies on preprocedural imaging studies versus final pathologic evaluation.

Dowlatshahi and colleagues[57] have also recently reported the results of interstitial laser ablation in 2 patients who had 3 breast fibroadenomas treated. Laser ablation produced coagulation of the tumor and a rim of surrounding normal breast tissue, which liquefied over time. Tumor shrinkage was observed on follow-up imaging, forming a scar. The investigators concluded that interstitial laser therapy could serve as an alternative to surgical excision for benign breast tumors.

In addition to mammography, ultrasonography and MRI have also been used to guide interstitial laser ablation therapy.[53,58,59] MRI has been used as the image-guidance modality during interstitial laser thermotherapy for liver tumors. Its utility resides in the fact that real-time tissue necrosis can be observed and real-time tissue temperature can be monitored, and adjustments in the delivery of therapy can be made.[59,60] MRI-guided laser ablation has also been used in the context of a clinical protocol as a palliative therapy for patients with Stage IV breast cancer.[59]

High-Intensity Focused Ultrasound Therapy

High-intensity focused ultrasound therapy is a completely noninvasive thermal therapy that has been studied in the ablation of breast fibroadenomas and carcinomas. This treatment modality applies focused ultrasound waves to a tumor transcutaneously, thus eliminating the need for skin entry as is needed in other ablative therapies.[61,62] The high temperatures used in ultrasound therapy cause a rapid melting of the lipid bilayer in cellular membranes and protein denaturation, producing tissue necrosis.[36]

The technique of high-intensity focused ultrasound ablation may be performed in the outpatient setting under conscious sedation. The tumor to be treated must be visible on ultrasonography, with clearly defined margins. Also, there cannot be any important bodily structures within the ultrasound beam pathway, so that target localization through an acoustic window on the skin can occur.[61] The tumor must be located at a distance of 1 cm deep to the skin surface to avoid thermal injury, as well as 1 cm from the chest wall to avoid injury to the underlying ribs and lung.[63] Either ultrasound imaging or MRI can be used for image guidance and tumor localization during the ablation. The patient is placed in the supine position for treatment if ultrasound guidance is to be used, or in the prone position with the breast immobilized if MRI guidance is used.[63–67] A coupling gel is applied to the patient's skin, and an extracorporeal transducer is positioned on the patient's skin overlying the tumor. The transducer serves as the energy source and generates ultrasonic beams that propagate through the breast tissue as high-frequency pressure waves and meet focally in the tumor where they will be absorbed. Ultrasound ablation is performed at this focal point (**Fig. 9**).[62,63] Ultrasound beam frequencies in the range of 0.5 to 4.0 MHz are used, depending on the depth of penetration that is required.[63] The pressure fluctuations that occur within the tissue cause shearing at a microscopic level, which produces frictional heating and thermal coagulation.[61,63] A temperature of 56°C or more must be achieved and maintained for at least 1 second in the target tissue to allow coagulation necrosis and cell death to occur.[61–64] The amount of cellular destruction that occurs is determined by the end temperature within the tissue and the length of time it is maintained.[62,63] Breast tissue that is within the propagation path of the ultrasound beams, but outside the focal point, is unaffected.[61,62] If a large lesion or multiple lesions are to be ultrasonically ablated, the transducer may be moved to change the focal point as necessary.[61]

Hynynen and colleagues[65] have studied this ablative therapy in the treatment of patients with benign breast tumors. Nine patients with 11 biopsy-proven fibroadenomas underwent MRI-guided ultrasound ablation. Patients did not undergo surgical resection after the ultrasound ablation. Adverse effects that were cited include postprocedure edema in 1 patient, bruising in 1 patient, and mild pain in 4 patients. Eight of 11 tumors showed partial or complete lack of contrast uptake on postprocedural MRI, implying tissue devascularization and tumor necrosis. For the remaining 3 patients who did not have successful ablation based on the MRI appearance, low acoustic power or patient movement were cited as the reasons for therapy failure. Thus, the investigators concluded that MRI-guided ultrasound ablation was feasible and safe in the treatment of breast fibroadenomas.

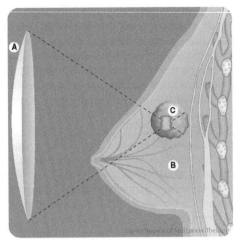

Fig. 9. The principle of high-intensity focused ultrasonography for tumor ablation. Ultrasound energy is focused into a small volume in which it is converted into heat to induce the required thermal ablation of a targeted breast tumor. A, high-intensity focused ultrasound transducer; B, normal breast tissue; C, the targeted breast tumor at the focal point. *(Reprinted from* Wu F, ter Haar G, Cen WR. High-intensity focused ultrasound ablation of breast cancer. Expert Rev Anticancer Ther 2007;7:825; Copyright 2007, with permission from Expert Reviews Ltd.)

This ablative modality has also been evaluated in the treatment of patients with breast cancer by Wu and colleagues.[64] Twenty-three patients with tumors 4.7 cm or smaller (21 with invasive cancer, 2 with noninvasive cancer) were treated with ultrasound-guided high-intensity focused ultrasound ablation. Ultrasound ablation was followed by modified radical mastectomy within 2 weeks of their ablative therapy. Side effects of the treatment included edema, breast heaviness, mild pain, and mild skin burn. On histologic evaluation, complete coagulation necrosis was observed in the tumors of all 23 patients, along with pyknotic nuclei and nuclear disruption, indicating that cell death had occurred. To ensure complete destruction of the breast cancer with negative margins, the investigators advocated ablating a margin of 1.5 to 2.0 cm of healthy-appearing tissue at the periphery of the tumor.

MRI-guided high-intensity focused ultrasound ablation has also been evaluated without resection in patients with significant comorbidities that preclude surgery. Gianfelice and colleagues[67] treated 24 patients with breast cancers 2.5 cm or less in size with ultrasound ablation without surgical resection. Sixteen of these 24 patients were considered high risk for surgical intervention because of the presence of significant comorbidities, while 8 patients refused surgery. All 24 patients were receiving tamoxifen therapy. Twenty-three of the 24 patients completed the planned ablative therapy. After ablation, patients were followed with core-needle biopsies and contrast-enhanced MRI. Out of 23 patients who completed the planned ablative therapy, 19 had negative postprocedure biopsies at a mean follow-up of 20.2 months. Eighteen of these 19 patients had no contrast enhancement on follow-up MRI, indicating tumor destruction. The investigators proposed that ultrasound ablation may be considered for local disease control in patients who are not surgical candidates.

Similar to what has been observed with cryoablation, high-intensity focused ultrasound ablation has also been reported to activate the immune system. Xu and colleagues[68] studied the surgical resection specimens of 23 women with breast cancer who underwent high-intensity focused ultrasound ablation followed by modified radical mastectomy. Immunohistochemical staining revealed the presence of antigen-presenting cells infiltrating the margins of the ablated regions along with the activation of dendritic cells and macrophages. Further studies will be necessary to determine whether ultrasound ablation therapy stimulates a systemic antitumor immunologic response that could be beneficial in reducing rates of local-regional recurrence and distant metastases.[63,68]

In contrast to other ablative approaches described in this article, an additional advantage of high-intensity focused ultrasound ablation is the completely noninvasive nature of this approach. Consequently, this technique is associated with less patient discomfort intraprocedurally and postprocedurally. Moreover, cosmetic results are improved because there is no scarring at a skin entry site. As advancements in imaging, energy delivery techniques, and margin delineation occur, protocols evaluating the clinical applicability of high-intensity focused ultrasound ablation for local disease control will expand.[61,63]

Focused Microwave Therapy

Focused microwave ablation is a minimally invasive approach that may be well suited for the treatment of early-stage breast cancers because microwave energy preferentially heats and destroys tissue with a high water content, such as breast tumors.[69–71] The technique uses electromagnetic waves at frequencies of 900 MHz or greater to generate heat, resulting in tumor destruction.[72] Advantages of this therapy include high intratumoral temperatures, the ability to generate a large treatment field, fast treatment times, and the ability to conduct multiple ablations simultaneously.[72] Because focused microwave ablation does not require an electrical current to pass through the patient's body as other hyperthermic ablative therapies do, the use of grounding pads is not necessary, thus skin burns at remote sites do not occur.[72] In the ablation of liver tumors, microwave therapy has been reported to destroy tissue up to 2 cm from the probe site, producing a uniform zone of ablation and tumor destruction.[72]

An electric-field probe is inserted under ultrasound guidance into the central portion of the tumor to focus the microwaves and to monitor microwave field amplitude during the ablation. In a similar fashion, a fiber-optic temperature probe is placed into the tumor to guide and adjust the thermotherapy to the desired temperature. Noninvasive temperature probes may also be applied to the surface of the skin to monitor therapy.[69] Compression of the breast is helpful for multiple reasons: it minimizes movement of the treatment field, reduces the depth of penetration needed, decreases blood flow to the tumor, and increases the efficiency of microwave energy transfer. A cooling system should also be employed, such as an external fan directing air at the patient's breast, to decrease the risk of thermal injury to the skin during the ablative treatment (**Fig. 10**).[69]

A pilot study to assess the feasibility and safety of focused microwave thermotherapy[69] was performed in 10 patients with breast cancers ranging in size from 1.0 to 8.0 cm. The tumors were ablated with a 915-MHz focused microwave thermotherapy system with a mean peak tumor temperature of 44.9°C. Surgical resection was performed 5 to 27 days after ablation. Complications of the microwave ablation included skin necrosis and blistering. Postprocedural ultrasound imaging demonstrated a reduction in tumor size in 6 of the 10 patients who were treated. On evaluation of the resection specimens, tumor cell kill was evident in 7 patients. However, no patients showed evidence of complete tumor cell kill. It would be of interest to know whether the size of the tumor correlated with the percentage of necrosis or apoptosis;

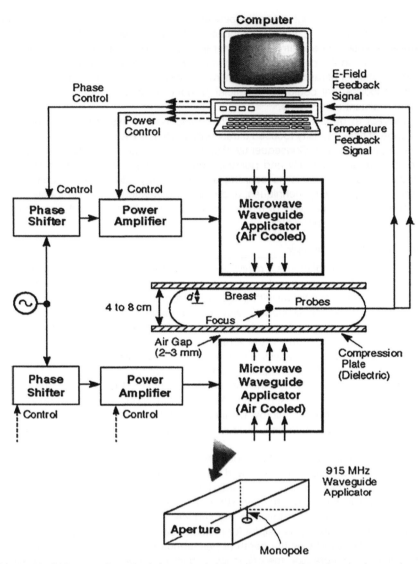

Fig. 10. Block diagram for a dual-channel adaptive microwave phased-array thermotherapy system for treating breast cancer. The breast-compression plates are made of an acrylic material transparent to microwaves. Air cooling through the rectangular waveguide applicators is used to reduce the skin temperatures. The applicators generate a focused electric-field radiation pattern that will illuminate a large volume of breast tissue. High-water content breast carcinomas may heat more rapidly than the surrounding normal breast tissues when exposed to the microwave field. (*From* Gardner RA, Vargas HI, Block JB, et al. Focused microwave phased array thermotherapy for primary breast cancer. Ann Surg Oncol 2002;9:327; with permission from Springer Science & Business Media and Robert A. Gardner, MD.)

however, this information is not provided. The investigators propose that focused microwave thermotherapy could potentially be used to downsize breast tumors, making breast conservation a possibility for some patients who initially had large tumors or an unfavorable tumor-to-breast ratio.[69]

Vargas and colleagues[70] conducted a prospective, multicenter, phase 2 study to determine the minimum thermal dose that was safe and effective in producing a complete tumor kill of breast carcinoma. Using a 915-MHz focused microwave thermotherapy system, 25 patients with tumor diameters ranging from 0.7 to 2.8 cm were treated. Although pathologic evaluation showed some degree of necrosis in 17 patients, complete necrosis of invasive carcinoma was achieved in only 2 patients. Tumor necrosis was related to the thermal energy dose delivered and peak tumor temperature achieved. In this study, a thermal dose of 210 cumulative equivalent minutes and a peak temperature of 49.7°C were required for complete tumor destruction.

Vargas and colleagues[73] also evaluated the feasibility of performing sentinel lymph node biopsy after focused microwave thermotherapy in women with breast cancer. Twenty-one patients with T1-T2 invasive cancers and a clinically negative axilla underwent microwave ablation followed by sentinel lymph node dissection at the time of their surgical resection, between 6 and 38 days after the ablation. Sentinel lymph node mapping was performed with peritumoral injections of blue dye and technetium sulfur colloid, and was successful in 19 patients (91%). Although this study shows that sentinel lymph node mapping was feasible after microwave ablation, the issue of accuracy still remains because all patients did not have a completion axillary lymph node dissection to confirm the results of their sentinel lymph node biopsy.[73]

Focused microwave thermotherapy shares similar advantages and disadvantages to other minimally invasive ablative therapies. However, there may be more patient discomfort with this approach than with others, due to the prone position that is recommended for optimal breast compression. To date, microwave thermotherapy has not been evaluated in any large prospective randomized trials.[71]

SUMMARY

Ablative therapies are a minimally invasive form of treatment for benign and malignant breast disease that have several potential advantages over standard surgical resection. These treatments can usually be performed in an ambulatory setting without the use of general anesthesia, resulting in increased convenience and decreased costs. These therapies produce cosmetically appealing results, as there is minimal change to the contour of the breast because no tissue resection occurs; thus, there is no volume loss. Also, in patients who cannot undergo formal surgical resection or general anesthesia because of medical comorbidities, percutaneous ablative therapies offer an opportunity for treatment.

Areas of ongoing controversy include the timing of sentinel lymph node biopsy and appropriate imaging follow-up after ablative therapy. Delayed contrast-enhanced MRI may be superior to other imaging modalities, due to its ability to visualize the devascularized treated regions as areas of nonenhancement.[61,70]

The feasibility of these various ablative techniques has been demonstrated for benign breast fibroadenomas. However, prospective controlled multi-institutional trials, such as the ACOSOG Z1072 study for cryoablation, are needed to establish their role in the treatment of breast carcinoma.

REFERENCES

1. Fisher B, Jeong J, Anderson S, et al. Twenty-five-year follow-up of a randomized trial comparing radical mastectomy, total mastectomy, and total mastectomy followed by irradiation. N Engl J Med 2002;347:567–75.

2. Fisher B, Anderson S, Bryant J, et al. Twenty-year follow-up of a randomized trial comparing total mastectomy, lumpectomy, and lumpectomy plus irradiation for the treatment of invasive breast cancer. N Engl J Med 2002;347:1233–41.

3. Veronesi U, Cascinelli N, Mariani L, et al. Twenty-year follow-up of a randomized study comparing breast-conserving surgery with radical mastectomy for early breast cancer. N Engl J Med 2002;347:1227–32.

4. Lyman GH, Giuliano AE, Somerfield MR, et al. American Society of Clinical Oncology guideline recommendations for sentinel lymph node biopsy in early-stage breast cancer. J Clin Oncol 2005;23(30):7703–20.

5. Krag DN, Anderson SJ, Julian TB, et al. Technical outcomes of sentinel-lymph-node resection and conventional axillary node-negative breast cancer: results from the NSABP B-32 randomised phase III trial. Lancet Oncol 2007;8:881.

6. Mansel RE, Fallowfield L, Kissin M, et al. Randomized multicenter trial of sentinel node biopsy versus standard axillary treatment in operable breast cancer: the ALMANAC Trial. J Natl Cancer Inst 2006;98:599.

7. Gillams AR. The use of radiofrequency in cancer. Br J Cancer 2005;92:1825–9.

8. Mirza AN, Fornage BD, Sneige N, et al. Radiofrequency ablation of solid tumors. Cancer J Sci Am 2001;7:95–102.

9. van der Ploeg IM, van Esser S, van den Bosch MA, et al. Radiofrequency ablation for breast cancer: a review of the literature. Eur J Surg Oncol 2007;33:673–7.

10. van Esser S, van den Bosch MA, van Diest PJ, et al. Minimally invasive ablative therapies for invasive breast carcinomas: an overview of the current literature. World J Surg 2007;31:2284–92.

11. Singeltary SE. Minimally invasive ablation techniques in breast cancer treatment. Ann Surg Oncol 2002;9:319–20.

12. Singeltary SE. Feasibility of radiofrequency ablation for primary breast cancer. Breast Cancer 2003;10:4–9.

13. Jeffrey SS, Birdwell RL, Ikeda DM, et al. Radiofrequency ablation of breast cancer: first report on emerging technology. Arch Surg 1999;134:1064–8.

14. Fornage BD, Sneige N, Ross MI, et al. Small (≤2 cm) breast cancer treated with us-guided radiofrequency ablation: feasibility study. Radiology 2004;231:215–24.

15. Medina-Franco H, Soto-Germes S, Uloa-Gomez JL, et al. Radiofrequency ablation of invasive breast carcinomas a phase II trial. Ann Surg Oncol 2008;15:1689–95.

16. Izzo F, Thomas R, Delerio P, et al. Radiofrequency ablation in patients with primary breast carcinoma: a pilot study in 26 patients. Cancer 2001;92:2036–44.

17. Imoto S, Wada N, Sakemura N, et al. Feasibility study on radiofrequency ablation followed by partial mastectomy for stage I breast cancer patients. Breast 2009; 18:130–4.

18. Manenti G, Bolacchi F, Perretta T, et al. Small breast cancers: in vivo percutaneous US-guided radiofrequency ablation with dedicated cool-tip radiofrequency system. Radiology 2009;251:339–46.

19. Head JF, Elliott RL, et al. Stereotactic radiofrequency ablation: a minimally invasive technique for nonpalpable breast cancer in postmenopausal patients. Cancer Epidemiol 2009;33:300–5.

20. Oura A, Tamaki T, Yoshimasu T, et al. Radiofrequency ablation therapy in patients with breast cancers two centimeters or less in size. Breast Cancer 2007;14:48–54.

21. Susini T, Nori J, Olivieri S, et al. Radiofrequency ablation for minimally invasive treatment of breast carcinoma. A pilot study in elderly inoperable patients. Gynecol Oncol 2006;104:304–10.

22. Yamamoto N, Fujimoto H, Nakamura R, et al. Pilot study of radiofrequency ablation therapy without surgical excision for T1 breast cancer: evaluation with MRI

and vacuum-assisted core needle biopsy and safety management. Breast Cancer 2010.

23. Klimberg VS, Kepple J, Shafirstein G, et al. eRFA: excision followed by RFA-a new technique to improve local control in breast cancer. Ann Surg Oncol 2006;13: 1422–33.

24. Ravikumar TS. The role of cryotherapy in the management of patients with liver tumors. Adv Surg 1996;30:281–91.

25. Baust JG, Gage AA, Klossner D, et al. Issues critical to the successful application of cryosurgical ablation of the prostate. Technol Cancer Res Treat 2007;6:97–109.

26. Uchida M, Imaide Y, Sugimoto K, et al. Percutaneous cryosurgery for renal tumors. Br J Urol 1995;75:132–6.

27. Hoffmann NE, Bischof JC. The cryobiology of cryosurgical injury. Urology 2002; 60:40–9.

28. Sabel MS, Su G, Griffith KA, et al. Rate of freeze alters the immunologic response after cryoablation of breast cancer. Ann Surg Oncol 2010;17:1187–93.

29. Rewcastle JC, Sandison GA, Muldrew K, et al. A model for the time dependent three-dimensional thermal distribution within iceballs surrounding multiple cryo-probes. Med Phys 2001;28:1125–37.

30. Morin J, Traore A, Dionne G, et al. Magnetic resonance-guided percutaneous cryosurgery of breast carcinoma: technique and early clinical results. Can J Surg 2004;47:347–51.

31. Larson TR, Robertson DW, Corica A, et al. In vivo interstitial temperature mapping of the human prostate during cryosurgery with correlation to histopathologic outcomes. Urology 2000;55:547–52.

32. Littrup PJ, Freeman-Gibb L, Andea A, et al. Cryotherapy for breast fibroadeno-mas. Radiology 2005;234:63–72.

33. Sabel MS, Kaufman CS, Whitworth P, et al. Cryoablation of early-stage breast cancer: work-in progress report of a multi-institutional trial. Ann Surg Oncol 2004;11:542–9.

34. Reiser M, Drukier AK, Ultsch B, et al. The use of CT in monitoring cryosurgery. Eur J Radiol 1983;3:123–8.

35. Ching CD, Hunt KK. Percutaneous ablation: minimally invasive techniques in breast cancer therapy. In: Bland KI, Copeland EM, editors. The breast: compre-hensive management of benign and malignant diseases. 4th edition. Philadel-phia: Saunders (Elsevier); 2009. p. 1043–50.

36. Whitworth PW, Rewcastle JC. Cryoablation and cryolocalization in the manage-ment of breast disease. J Surg Onc 2005;90:1–9.

37. Sahoo S, Talwalkar SS, Martin AW, et al. Pathologic evaluation of cryoprobe-as-sisted lumpectomy for breast cancer. Am J Pathol 2007;128:239–44.

38. Pfleiderer SO, Freesmeyer MG, Marx C, et al. Cryotherapy of breast cancer under ultrasound guidance: initial results and limitations. Eur Radiol 2002;12:3009–14.

39. Rui J, Tatsutani KN, Dahiya R, et al. Effect of thermal variables on human breast cancer in cryosurgery. Breast Cancer Res Treat 1999;53:185–92.

40. Gage AA, Baust J. Mechanisms of tissue injury in cryosurgery. Cryobiology 1998; 37:171–86.

41. Nurko J, Mabry CD, Whitworth P, et al. Interim results from the FibroAdenoma Cryoablation Treatment Registry. Am J Surg 2005;190:647–51.

42. Sabel MS, Nehs MA, Su G, et al. Immunologic response to cryoablation of breast cancer. Breast Cancer Res Treat 2005;90:97–104.

43. Pfleiderer SO, Marx C, Camara O, et al. Ultrasound-guided, percutaneous cryo-therapy of small (≤15 mm) breast cancers. Invest Radiol 2005;40:472–7.

44. Kaufman CS, Littrup PJ, Freeman-Gibb LA, et al. Office-based cryoablation of breast fibroadenomas with long-term follow-up. Breast J 2005;11:344–50.
45. Tafra L, Fine R, Whitworth P, et al. Prospective randomized study comparing cryo-assisted and needle-wire localization of ultrasound-visible breast tumors. Am J Surg 2006;192:462–70.
46. Rand RW. Cryolumpectomy for carcinoma of the breast. Surg Gynecol Obstet 1987;165:392–6.
47. Suzuki Y. Cryosurgical treatment of advanced breast cancer and cryoimmunological responses. Skin Cancer 1995;10:19–26.
48. Tanaka S. Cryosurgical treatment of advanced breast cancer. Skin Cancer 1995; 10:9–18.
49. National Cancer Institute Clinical Trials PDQ. Phase II study of cryoablation therapy in patients with invasive ductal breast carcinoma. Available at: http://www.cancer.gov/clinicaltrials/ACOSOG-Z1072. Assessed June 21, 2010.
50. National Institutes of Health ClinicalTrials.gov. Cryoablation therapy in treating patients with invasive ductal breast cancer. Available at: http://clinicaltrials.gov/ct2/show/NCT00723294. Assessed June 21, 2010.
51. Dowlatshahi K, Fan M, Gould VE, et al. Stereotactically guided laser therapy of occult breast tumors: work-in-progress report. Arch Surg 2000;135:1345–52.
52. Shafirstein G, Novak P, Moros EG, et al. Conductive interstitial thermal therapy device for surgical margin ablation: in vivo verification of a theoretical model. Int J Hyperthermia 2007;23:477–92.
53. van Esser S, Stapper G, van Diest PJ, et al. Ultrasound-guided laser-induced thermal therapy for small palpable invasive breast carcinomas: a feasibility study. Ann Surg Oncol 2009;16:2259–63.
54. Milne PJ, Parel JM, Manns F, et al. Development of stereotactically guided laser interstitial thermotherapy of breast cancer: in situ measurement and analysis of the temperature field in ex vivo and in vivo adipose tissue. Lasers Surg Med 2000;26:67–75.
55. Robinson DS, Parel JM, Denham DB, et al. Interstitial laser hyperthermia model development for minimally invasive therapy of breast carcinoma. J Am Coll Surg 1998;186:284–92.
56. Dowlatshahi K, Francescatti DS, Bloom KJ. Laser therapy for small breast cancers. Am J Surg 2002;184:359–63.
57. Dowlatshahi K, Wadhwani S, Alvarado R, et al. Interstitial laser therapy of breast fibroadenomas with 6 and 8 year follow-up. Breast J 2010;16:73–6.
58. Haraldsdottir KH, Ivarsson K, Gotberg S, et al. Interstitial laser thermotherapy (ILT) of breast cancer. Eur J Surg Oncol 2008;34:739–45.
59. Akimov AB, Seregin VE, Rusanov KV, et al. Nd:YAG Interstitial laser thermotherapy in the treatment of breast cancer. Lasers Surg Med 1998;22:257–67.
60. Vogl TJ, Straub R, Zangos S, et al. MR-guided laser-induced thermotherapy (LITT) of liver tumors: experimental and clinical data. Int J Hyperthermia 2004;20:713–24.
61. Haar GT, Coussios C. High intensity focused ultrasound: physical principles and devices. Int J Hyperthermia 2007;23:89–104.
62. Wu F, Haar GT, Chen WR. High-intensity focused ultrasound ablation of breast cancer. Expert Rev Anticancer Ther 2007;7:823–31.
63. Schmitz AC, Gianfelice D, Daniel BL, et al. Image-guided focused ultrasound ablation of breast cancer: current status, challenges, and future directions. Eur Radiol 2008;18:1431–41.
64. Wu F, Wang ZB, Cao YD, et al. "Wide local ablation" of localized breast cancer using high intensity focused ultrasound. J Surg Oncol 2007;96:130–6.

65. Hynynen K, Pomeroy O, Smith DN, et al. MR imaging-guided focused ultrasound surgery of fibroadenomas in the breast: a feasibility study. Radiology 2001;219: 176–85.
66. Furusawa H, Namba K, Nakahara H, et al. The evolving non-surgical ablation of breast cancer: MR guided focused ultrasound (MRgFUS). Breast Cancer 2007; 14(1):55–8.
67. Gianfelice D, Khiat A, Boulanger Y, et al. Feasibility of magnetic resonance imaging-guided focused ultrasound surgery as an adjunct to Tamoxifen therapy in high-risk surgical patients with breast carcinoma. J Vasc Interv Radiol 2003;14: 1275–82.
68. Xu ZL, Zhu XQ, Lu P, et al. Activation of tumor-infiltrating antigen presenting cells by high intensity focused ultrasound ablation of human breast cancer. Ultrasound Med Biol 2009;35:50–7.
69. Gardner RA, Vargas HI, Block JB, et al. Focused microwave phased array thermotherapy for primary breast cancer. Ann Surg Oncol 2002;9:326–32.
70. Vargas HI, Dooley WC, Gardner RA, et al. Focused microwave phased array thermotherapy for ablation of early-stage breast cancer: results of thermal dose escalation. Ann Surg Oncol 2004;11:139–46.
71. Dooley WC, Vargas HI, Fenn AJ, et al. Focused microwave thermotherapy for preoperative treatment of invasive breast cancer: a review of clinical studies. Ann Surg Oncol 2010;17:1076–93.
72. Martin RC, Scoggins CR, McMasters KM. Microwave hepatic ablation: initial experience of safety and efficacy. J Surg Oncol 2007;96:481–6.
73. Vargas HI, Dooley WC, Gardner RA, et al. Success of sentinel lymph node mapping after breast cancer ablation with focused microwave phased array thermotherapy. Am J Surg 2003;186:330–2.

Ablation of Kidney Tumors

Jose A. Karam, MD[a], Kamran Ahrar, MD[b,c],
Surena F. Matin, MD[a,d],*

KEYWORDS

- Renal mass • Kidney cancer • Renal cell carcinoma
- Radiofrequency ablation • Catheter-ablation • Cryoablation
- Survival • Complications

The American Cancer Society estimates that more than 50,000 patients in the United States are diagnosed with renal malignancies each year and that 10,000 of these patients will die of their disease.[1] Most renal malignancies are low-stage, low-grade renal cell carcinomas.[2] Recently, diagnoses of small renal cell carcinomas have increased, especially among patients older than 70 years,[3,4] in part because of the widespread use of abdominal ultrasonography and computed tomography (CT). Most renal cell carcinomas are detected incidentally.[5–8]

Radical nephrectomy, once the primary treatment of small renal cell carcinoma, has been associated with a relatively high incidence of chronic kidney disease, cardiovascular mortality, and overall mortality, and is now considered overtreatment. Today, the standard of care for most patients with small renal cell carcinoma is surgical extirpation by partial nephrectomy, which provides disease control equivalent to that of radical nephrectomy but with the advantage of renal preservation[9–13] However, some patients with small renal cell carcinomas, including elderly patients and patients with renal dysfunction are poor candidates for surgical extirpation. For these patients, radiofrequency ablation (RFA) or cryoablation may be a more appropriate treatment option.

The University of Texas MD Anderson Cancer Center is supported in part by the National Institutes of Health through Cancer Center Support Grant CA 016672.
The authors have nothing to disclose.
[a] Department of Urology, The University of Texas MD Anderson Cancer Center, Unit 1373, 1515 Holcombe Boulevard, Houston, TX 77030, USA
[b] Department of Diagnostic Imaging, The University of Texas MD Anderson Cancer Center, Unit 0325, 1515 Holcombe Boulevard, Houston, TX 77030, USA
[c] Section of Interventional Radiology, The University of Texas MD Anderson Cancer Center, Unit 0325, 1515 Holcombe Boulevard, Houston, TX 77030, USA
[d] Minimally Invasive New Technology in Oncologic Surgery (MINTOS), The University of Texas MD Anderson Cancer Center, Unit 1373, 1515 Holcombe Boulevard, Houston, TX 77030, USA
* Corresponding author. Department of Urology, The University of Texas MD Anderson Cancer Center, Unit 1373, 1515 Holcombe Boulevard, Houston, TX 77030.
E-mail address: surmatin@mdanderson.org

Patients who qualify for ablative therapy should be considered to first have a biopsy of the renal mass for histologic confirmation of malignancy. Those confirmed to have a benign tumor may be counseled to only undergo surveillance. Patients need to be made aware of therapeutic alternatives, potential complications, need for strict imaging surveillance for an indefinite period of time, and the potential need for post-ablation biopsy to histologically confirm treatment success. Patients who are unable to meet these criteria should not be considered for ablative therapy.

RADIOFREQUENCY ABLATION
Mechanism of Action

In RFA, heat is generated by friction of water molecules reacting to radiofrequencies, and the heat destroys tumor tissue. Ex vivo and in vivo RFA of renal tumors was initially described by Zlotta and colleagues[14] in 1997; since then, the use of RFA for treating renal masses has surged. Hsu and colleagues[15] used light microscopy and a porcine model to study RFA-induced histologic changes in the renal parenchyma and found that chromatin blurring, increased cytoplasmic eosinophilia, loss of cell membrane integrity, and interstitial hemorrhage were among the earliest changes following RFA. Three days after RFA, Hsu and colleagues[15] noted extensive coagulative necrosis with early infiltration of fibroblasts and acute inflammatory elements at the border of the RFA. At 1 week, nuclear degeneration was more pronounced, and acute inflammatory elements had increased. At 2 weeks, nuclear degeneration was complete; and at 4 weeks, loss of cytoplasmic borders and features characteristic of renal parenchyma were present. Renal parenchyma 1 cm from the ablation zone appeared histologically normal. At 3 months, near-total resorption of the lesion had occurred.

Cell death resulting from RFA begins after 5 minutes of exposure to temperatures at or more than 50°C. However, temperatures greater than 105°C are counterproductive because they cause acute tissue vaporization and eschar formation that limits heat conduction and thus the efficacy of RFA. For effective thermal ablation, homogeneous RFA electrode temperatures in the range of 50°C to 100°C must be maintained throughout the target area.[16] Multitined probes, saline-cooled probes, temperature or impedance monitoring, and other mechanisms are used by various manufacturers to maintain ideal temperatures.

Technique

At our institution, we typically perform a core needle biopsy of the renal mass using a 20-gauge coaxial needle to confirm malignant histology before performing RFA. After renal cell carcinoma is confirmed by permanent section analysis, RFA can then be performed percutaneously under CT guidance or laparoscopically under direct visualization and intraoperative ultrasonography guidance.

The percutaneous RFA technique that we use has been described in detail previously but is briefly reviewed here.[17] Percutaneous RFA is performed with the patient under general anesthesia. We and others[18] believe that general anesthesia is key to localizing and targeting small renal masses accurately; other investigators prefer using intravenous sedation.[19,20] The patient is placed in the prone position, and CT is used to localize the tumor. Ablation is performed using a 200-W impedance-based device. One or more electrodes are positioned in the tumor under CT guidance. Then, sequential overlapping ablations are performed as indicated by the size and location of the tumor until the tumor is completely ablated.

In patients in whom the renal lesion and colon are in proximity to one another, hydro-dissection is performed by injecting saline in a plane between the kidney and colon to improve the safety of RFA.[21] Similarly, cooled saline can be injected in a retrograde fashion through the ureter to protect it from heat damage.[20,22,23] Additional maneuvers to safely target the lesion include torquing the RFA probe manually and positioning an angioplasty balloon between the tumor and bowel.[21]

Immediately after RFA, intravenous contrast material can be administered to assess the ablation zone and adequate ablation of the lesion.

Lesions that cannot be safely treated by percutaneous RFA, such as anterior tumors and tumors close to the renal hilum or ureter, can be treated with transperitoneal lapa-roscopic RFA. To avoid damage to the renal hilum, ureter, or adjacent normal struc-tures, transperitoneal laparoscopic RFA is performed with the patient under general anesthesia. The patient is placed in the modified flank position. A Veress needle is used to access the peritoneum, 3 laparoscopic ports are placed, the colon is mobi-lized medially, the kidney is identified, and the ureter mobilized away from the treat-ment area if necessary. Perinephric fat (except for the fat in immediate contact with the tumor) is mobilized away from the kidney. Intraoperative ultrasonography is then used to assess the extent of the tumor and the tumor's relation to adjacent structures.

Before ablation is performed, small cautery marks that will serve as visual landmarks to aid in repositioning the probe are made at the margin of the proposed treatment zone. This is done because as treatment proceeds, the lesion contracts and anatomic landmarks become subtle or disappear on ultrasonography. The RFA probe is then inserted into the tumor under ultrasound guidance until the probe tip is at or just past the deepest tumor-renal parenchyma interface. Optimal initial probe targeting is key; as RFA starts, tissue vaporization and cavitation degrade the ultrasound image, diminishing accurate targeting capability. Treating the deepest margin first effectively achieves a vascular amputation such that subsequent, more superficial overlapping ablations can be completed more quickly. Ablation is performed using a 200-W impedance-controlled device following a standardized protocol. Each initial session is followed by a second confirmatory session, after which the ablation probe is partially withdrawn and another sequential ablation performed. The probe is repositioned as necessary, and the process is repeated until the entire tumor and margin are treated. The perirenal fat is then approximated with absorbable sutures, and a standard lapa-roscopic exit is performed.

CRYOABLATION
Mechanism of Action

Four thermal parameters are used to determine the rate of cellular damage during cry-oablation: cooling rate, minimum temperature reached, time maintained at the minimum temperature, and thawing rate.[24] Cryoablation directly kills tumor cells by causing osmotic dehydration that damages enzymatic pathways,[24,25] organelles, and the cell membrane and by causing intracellular ice formation that supercools the cytoplasmic contents.[24] Cryoablation also indirectly kills tumor cells by targeting small blood vessels,[26] which results in a hypoxic microenvironment[27] in which tumor cells cannot survive. To ensure adequate tumor treatment, a temperature of $-40°C$ must be achieved throughout the tumor; this typically occurs when the ice ball extends 0.5 to 1 cm beyond the tumor margins.[28]

The immunologic sequelae after cryoablation are interesting and potentially of clin-ical relevance. Recently, we investigated the immunologic sequelae of cryoablation in a murine model of renal cell carcinoma[29] and found increased lymphocytic infiltration in cryoablated lesions, especially in areas surrounding blood vessels and areas of sublethal tissue injury. Neutrophils, macrophages, and CD4+ and CD8+ T cells with an increased ratio of T helper type 1 cells to T helper type 2 cells were the most common immune reaction components. In addition, cryoablated lesions showed increased interferon-gamma production.[29] There is great interest in developing combinatorial strategies using cryoablation and immunotherapeutic modulation for treatment of metastatic renal cell carcinoma.[30]

Technique

Depending on the technology available, experience of the attending surgeon, and location and size of the tumor, cryoablation can be performed using an open, percutaneous, or laparoscopic approach. The laparoscopic approach is similar to that used for RFA, with the notable exception that ultrasound can and should be used throughout the freezing process to monitor the ice ball. Percutaneous cryoablation is performed similar to RFA as previously described. Cryoablation units use argon gas to achieve rapid freezing at the tip of the probe. The benefit of argon gas is that smaller-diameter probes can be used, and the ice ball formation terminates at the end of the freezing cycle.[31] As a result of the Joule-Thomson effect, depressurized argon gas has temperatures ranging from $-80°C$ to $-195°C$. Helium, which follows the reverse effect to release heat as it is depressurized, is thus used for the thawing cycle. Typically, 2 freeze/thaw cycles are performed, and multiple probes can be placed in the tumor if one probe is not sufficient to cover the entire tumor and its margin.[32,33] The ice ball is usually monitored using magnetic resonance imaging or CT fluoroscopy during percutaneous procedures and with a steerable laparoscopic ultrasonography probe during laparoscopic procedures.

FOLLOW-UP AND OUTCOMES AFTER ABLATIVE THERAPY

Routine follow-up after RFA includes medical history, physical examination, chest imaging with conventional radiography or CT, complete metabolic profiles, and other diagnostic tests for potential metastatic locations. We typically obtain contrast-enhanced CT or magnetic resonance images of the RFA lesion within 6 weeks of initial therapy, and then at 6, 12, 18, and 24 months.[34] Depending on the imaging study results, semiannual or annual follow-up is performed thereafter.

Definition of Local Treatment Success

Because the tumor is not excised after ablation and thus no tissue is available for histopathologic analysis, radiographic studies must be used to determine treatment success. Successful ablation is typically defined as a lack of enhancement after injection of intravenous contrast material and tumor involution. However, unlike lesions treated with cryoablation, RFA-treated lesions do not always involute, complicating the assessment of success, and reducing it to just absence of enhancement. Matsumoto and colleagues[35] studied the natural radiological history of 64 RFA-treated renal tumors and found that endophytic tumors developed a low-density, nonenhancing, wedge-shaped defect with fat infiltration between the ablated tissue and normal renal parenchyma, but that exophytic tumors retained a configuration similar to that of the original tumor with a lack of contrast enhancement and minimal involution.[35] However, in cases in which no enhancement and minimal involution were present, we found that biopsy of the ablation zones 6 months after RFA revealed viable tumor cells in about 10% of cases (data presented at Genitourinary Cancers Symposium, American Society of Clinical Oncology Annual Meeting 2010, San Francisco). Others have also reported finding viable cancer cells in the absence of contrast enhancement.[36] There can be not only false-negative imaging findings but also false-positive imaging findings can occur and alter clinical management.[37] Therefore, if ablation zones increase in size or fail to involute even in the absence of contrast enhancement 6 months after the initial ablation, we routinely obtain multiquadrant core biopsy specimens. The potential need for biopsy after ablation should be discussed with the patient, who must accept it as part of the treatment plan even before ablative therapy is initiated.

Functional Outcomes

Ablative therapy seems to cause less renal function loss than partial nephrectomy and certainly much less than radical nephrectomy. Lucas and colleagues[38] used the Modification of Diet in Renal Disease equation to compare renal function in patients who underwent RFA, partial nephrectomy, or radical nephrectomy and found that the rate of 3-year freedom from stage 3 chronic kidney disease (a decrease in glomerular filtration rate [GFR] of <60 mL/min/1.73 m^2) was 95.2% in patients who underwent RFA, 70.7% in patients who underwent partial nephrectomy, and 39.9% in patients who underwent radical nephrectomy ($P<.001$).

In a multi-institutional study, Raman and colleagues[39] evaluated renal function changes in patients with solitary kidneys and found that patients who underwent open partial nephrectomy under cold ischemic conditions had a greater decrease in GFR than patients who underwent RFA at all evaluated times, including soon after the procedure (15.8% vs 7.1%; $P<.001$), 12 months after the procedure (24.5% vs 10.4%; $P<.001$), and at last follow-up (28.6% vs 11.4%; $P<.001$). Weisbrod and colleagues[40] recently published the results of a large cohort of patients with solitary kidneys treated by percutaneous cryoablation, showing no patients needing dialysis and minimal change in GFR.

Differences Between Radiofrequency Ablation and Cryoablation

There are 2 key differences between cryoablation and RFA. First, in laparoscopic cryoablation, ultrasonography is eminently useful for monitoring the cryolesion; however, in laparoscopic RFA, ultrasonography cannot be used to effectively monitor the lesion because image quality starts to degrade as soon as treatment is initiated. Second, because multiple sequential treatments, which can be performed during RFA, cannot be performed during cryoablation, the initial geometric targeting by probe placement is critical in cryoablation. Biologic differences between the 2 modalities also probably exist, as RFA causes immediate vascular coagulation and thrombosis, whereas after cryoablation there is a period of vascular flow, vascular congestion, subsequently followed by thrombosis. This period of reestablished vasculature may provide greater exposure of tumor-associated antigens to immune cells.

Oncological Outcomes

The results of recent RFA and cryoablation series are summarized in **Tables 1** and **2**. Differences in reporting criteria and quality among studies should be noted when reviewing the ablation literature but can be difficult to discern. Definitions of incomplete ablation vary. The number of RFA sessions can vary, and success can be reported after the first, second, or third separate session. Some investigators report overall success regardless of the number of ablation sessions required. Because treatment success can be reported by measuring the rate of incomplete ablation, local recurrence at the site of ablation, recurrence in the contralateral kidney, or bona fide metastasis, success must be clearly defined when reporting the findings of these

Table 1
Results of RFA series as of 2005

Author, Year	No. of Patients	No. of Tumors	Mean Tumor Size, cm (Range)	Method	Mean Follow-up Time, Months (Range)	Local Recurrence/ Incomplete Ablation
Ahrar et al,[41] 2005	29	30	3.5 (SD, 0.2)	P	10 (1–33), median 7	1/24
Mahnken et al,[42] 2005	14	15	3 (SD, 1)	P	13.9 (SD 12.4)	0/15
Gervais et al,[20,23] 2005	85	100	3.2 (1.1–8.9)	P	27 (3–72)	9/85
Matsumoto et al,[43] 2005	91	109	2.4 (0.8–4.7)	P, L, O	19 (12–33)	3/91
Arzola et al,[44] 2006	23	27	2.7 (0.9–6)	P	24 (7–53)	4/20
Park et al,[45] 2006	78	94	2.4 (1–4.2)	P, L	25 (12–48)	5/94
Carey et al,[46] 2007	36	37	NR (3–5)	P, L	11.3 (1–44)	3/37
Stern et al,[47] 2007	40	40	2.4 (NR)	P, L	30 (18–42)	3/40
Breen et al,[48] 2007	97	105	3.2 (1.1–6.8)	P	18 (1–76)	22/105
Zagoria et al,[19] 2007	104	125	2.7 (0.6–8.8)	P	13.8 (1–76), median 9.8	16/125
Lucas et al,[38] 2008	86	86	2.3 (2.2–2.5)	P, L	Median 40 (NR)	6/86
Levinson et al,[49] 2008	31	31	2.1 (1–4)	P	61.6 (41–80), median 62	4/31
Wingo et al,[18] 2008	39	41	2.7 (1–5)	P, L	29 (NR)	4/41
Gupta et al,[18] 2009	151	163	2.3 (1–5.4)	P	18 (1.5–70)	5/163
Hoffmann et al,[50] 2010	10	13	2.7 (1.9–4.2)	P	NR (3–24)	0/13
Raman et al,[39] 2010	47	53	2.7 (1.5–6.5)	P, L	Median 18 (6–66)	5/47
Del Cura et al,[51] 2010	58	65	3.1 (1.2–5.3)	P	26.5 (10–50)	12/58

Abbreviations: L, laparoscopic; NR, not reported; O, open; P, percutaneous; SD, standard deviation.

Table 2
Results of cryoablation series as of 2005

Author, Year	No. of Patients	No. of Tumors	Mean Tumor Size, cm (Range)	Method	Mean Follow-up Time, Months (Range)	Local Recurrence/ Incomplete Ablation
Gill et al,[52] 2005	56	60	2.3 (1–5)	L	36 (NR)	2/56
Silverman et al,[53] 2005	23	26	2.6 (1–4.6)	P	14 (4–30)	3/23
Davol et al,[54] 2006	48	48	Median 2.6 (1.1–4.6)	O, L	Median 64 (36–110)	6/48
Gupta et al,[55] 2006	12	16	2.5 (1–4.6)	P	5.9 (NR)	1/12
Schwartz et al,[56] 2006	84	85	2.6 (1.2–4.7)	O, L	10 (3–36)	2/84
Miki et al,[57] 2006	13	13	2.7 (2–4.8)	P	35 (28–42)	2/13
Weld et al,[58] 2007	31	36	2.1 (0.5–4)	L	45.7 (NR)	1/31
Wyler et al,[59] 2007	14	14	2.8 (2–4)	O, L	21 (2–42)	0/14
Bandi et al,[60] 2007	78	88	1.6 (NR)	P, L	19 (2–62)	3/78
Atwell et al,[61] 2007	40	40	3.4 (1.5–7.2)	P	8 (1.2–18.4)	2/40
Atwell et al,[62] 2008	110	115	3.3 (1.5–7.3)	P	NR	3/110
Finley et al,[63] 2008	37	43	2.9 (1.1–5.4)	P, L	12.8 (2.7–34.7)	2/37
Malcolm et al,[64] 2009	66	72	2.3 (1–4.6)	P, L	Median 25, 30 (13–63)	7/66
Schmit et al,[65] 2010	108	110	4.1 (3–8.3)	P	15 (3–42)	3/108
Aron et al,[66] 2010	80	88	2.3 (0.9–5)	L	Median 93 (60–132)	4/80

Abbreviations: L, laparoscopic; NR, not reported; O, open; P, percutaneous.

studies. In addition, biopsies are not routinely performed before treatment and are performed even less frequently after treatment; the fact that about 25% of small renal masses are benign could confound reporting of recurrence or survival outcomes because a substantial number of patients may have had benign lesions to begin with. When biopsy results are available, outcomes should be stratified according to pathology findings. In addition, most studies report on success in terms of simple percentages without accounting for the fact that different patients are followed for different periods; the appropriate method would be to use a Kaplan-Meier plot, which accounts for patient censoring. Adding to the difficulties in evaluating the data is that the growth rate of small renal tumors may be very slow[67]; thus, in most patients the follow-up period is too short to draw definitive conclusions. These data deficiencies and limitations, which can also be attributed to much of the published literature on open surgery, were highlighted in the recent publication of the American Urological Associations Guidelines for Treatment of the Renal Mass.[68]

Predictors of Success

Gervais and colleagues[22] found that predictors of successful ablation included small tumor size and noncentral tumor location.[22] Breen and colleagues[48] also found small tumor size to be a predictor of successful RFA. Zagoria and colleagues[19] noted that a tumor diameter of less than 3.7 cm was significantly associated with complete tumor ablation and that the likelihood of tumor-free survival decreased by more than half with each 1-cm increase in tumor diameter more than 3.6 cm. In general, larger tumors (>3.5–4.5 cm, there is not perfect agreement on the size threshold), endophytic tumors (ie, tumors closer to the central sinus and larger vasculature), and more proximal tumor location are associated with higher rates of recurrence.[69,70] The disagreement about a size threshold is likely because this represents a continuum of risk rather than a categorical change in risk, and likely because it is additionally confounded by the location of tumors. A meta-analysis of the available literature revealed that ablative therapies have an oncologic effectiveness of 88% to 90% in the short and intermediate term, whereas open surgery has an efficacy of about 98%, even with long-term follow-up.[68]

COMPLICATIONS

Complications related to percutaneous probe access include pain, paresthesia, other neuromuscular complications, and pneumothorax at the sites of probe insertion and probe tract.[19,71,72] Bleeding after RFA is uncommon, occurring in less than 2% of patients.[19,20] Subclinical hematomas can occur and remain undetected; however, larger perirenal hematomas could manifest as flank pain, a decrease in hemoglobin levels, or alterations in vital signs. Typically, perirenal hematomas are managed with bed rest in the hospital, blood transfusions as necessary, and in refractory cases, selective angioembolization for optimal hemorrhage control. One particular complication after cryoablation is fracture of the ice ball, which results in potentially torrential, but usually self-limiting, hemorrhage on thawing.[68] This seems to be related to larger tumors and use of multiple probes.

With percutaneous RFA the tract can be cauterized with the RFA probe while it is being withdrawn from the mass to provide hemostatic control and to avoid track site seeding, a rare phenomenon that can be seen after ablative therapy and reported after cryoablation.[40] Occasionally, clots can occlude the ureter. In patients with a solitary kidney, renal failure necessitating dialysis can occur if the obstruction is not relieved quickly. These patients require temporary ureteral stenting until the clot resorbs. Bowel injuries are a rare event[73] and can be minimized by avoiding treatment of renal masses that are less than 1 cm away from bowel. Injury to the collecting system in the kidney, mainly the ureter/ureteropelvic junction, can occur,[71,73] and these patients need careful consideration of treatment of these lesions in close proximity to the collecting system.

SALVAGE THERAPY

Patients in whom disease recurs after initial thermal ablation require a full reevaluation with multiphasic contrast-enhanced dedicated renal imaging studies to assess the extent of the local recurrence and the presence or absence of regional and distant metastases. Salvage therapy can be performed[74,75] by repeat ablation with the same or different technology or with partial or radical nephrectomy. Typically, surgery after ablation is difficult because of extensive scarring and potential intraoperative complications, particularly in patients who have undergone laparoscopic cryoablation.[74] In our experience, salvage therapy in patients who have undergone percutaneous RFA is much more facile than in patients who have undergone laparoscopic cryoablation. This is likely related to the extensive laparoscopic mobilization that is performed at the time of cryoablation, and possibly related to the inflammatory reaction after cryoablation.

SUMMARY

Cryoablation and RFA are minimally invasive modalities that are well suited for treating small renal cell carcinomas in patients who cannot undergo definitive surgical excision. Data on the long-term efficacy of these therapies are forthcoming. Current meta-analyses suggest that cryoablation and RFA have efficacy that is reasonable at 88% to 90% with short- and intermediate-term follow-up, but not as good as that of surgical excision which is greater than 98% long-term. Patients who qualify for RFA or cryoablation should be made aware of therapeutic alternatives, potential complications, need for strict imaging surveillance for an indefinite period, and the potential need for biopsy to histologically confirm treatment success.

REFERENCES

1. Jemal A, Siegel R, Ward E, et al. Cancer statistics, 2009. CA Cancer J Clin 2009; 59(4):225–49.
2. Cohen HT, McGovern FJ. Renal-cell carcinoma. N Engl J Med 2005;353(23): 2477–90.
3. Chow WH, Devesa SS, Warren JL, et al. Rising incidence of renal cell cancer in the United States. JAMA 1999;281(17):1628–31.
4. Hollingsworth JM, Miller DC, Daignault S, et al. Rising incidence of small renal masses: a need to reassess treatment effect. J Natl Cancer Inst 2006;98(18): 1331–4.
5. Lightfoot N, Conlon M, Kreiger N, et al. Impact of noninvasive imaging on increased incidental detection of renal cell carcinoma. Eur Urol 2000;37(5): 521–7.
6. Luciani LG, Cestari R, Tallarigo C. Incidental renal cell carcinoma-age and stage characterization and clinical implications: study of 1092 patients (1982–1997). Urology 2000;56(1):58–62.
7. Bretheau D, Lechevallier E, Eghazarian C, et al. Prognostic significance of incidental renal cell carcinoma. Eur Urol 1995;27(4):319–23.

8. Jayson M, Sanders H. Increased incidence of serendipitously discovered renal cell carcinoma. Urology 1998;51(2):203–5.

9. Hafez KS, Fergany AF, Novick AC. Nephron sparing surgery for localized renal cell carcinoma: impact of tumor size on patient survival, tumor recurrence and TNM staging. J Urol 1999;162(6):1930–3.

10. Fergany AF, Hafez KS, Novick AC. Long-term results of nephron sparing surgery for localized renal cell carcinoma: 10-year followup. J Urol 2000;163(2):442–5.

11. Huang WC, Levey AS, Serio AM, et al. Chronic kidney disease after nephrectomy in patients with renal cortical tumours: a retrospective cohort study. Lancet Oncol 2006;7(9):735–40.

12. Weight CJ, Larson BT, Fergany AF, et al. Nephrectomy induced chronic renal insufficiency is associated with increased risk of cardiovascular death and death from any cause in patients with localized cT1b renal masses. J Urol 2010;183(4):1317–23.

13. Huang WC, Elkin EB, Levey AS, et al. Partial nephrectomy versus radical nephrectomy in patients with small renal tumors–is there a difference in mortality and cardiovascular outcomes? J Urol 2009;181(1):55–61 [discussion: 61–2].

14. Zlotta AR, Wildschutz T, Raviv G, et al. Radiofrequency interstitial tumor ablation (RITA) is a possible new modality for treatment of renal cancer: ex vivo and in vivo experience. J Endourol 1997;11(4):251–8.

15. Hsu TH, Fidler ME, Gill IS. Radiofrequency ablation of the kidney: acute and chronic histology in porcine model. Urology 2000;56(5):872–5.

16. Goldberg SN, Gazelle GS, Mueller PR. Thermal ablation therapy for focal malignancy: a unified approach to underlying principles, techniques, and diagnostic imaging guidance. AJR Am J Roentgenol 2000;174(2):323–31.

17. Jacobsohn KM, Ahrar K, Wood CG, et al. Is radiofrequency ablation safe for solitary kidneys? Urology 2007;69(5):819–23 [discussion: 823].

18. Gupta A, Raman JD, Leveillee RJ, et al. General anesthesia and contrast-enhanced computed tomography to optimize renal percutaneous radiofrequency ablation: multi-institutional intermediate-term results. J Endourol 2009;23(7):1099–105.

19. Zagoria RJ, Traver MA, Werle DM, et al. Oncologic efficacy of CT-guided percutaneous radiofrequency ablation of renal cell carcinomas. AJR Am J Roentgenol 2007;189(2):429–36.

20. Gervais DA, McGovern FJ, Arellano RS, et al. Radiofrequency ablation of renal cell carcinoma: part 1. Indications, results, and role in patient management over a 6-year period and ablation of 100 tumors. AJR Am J Roentgenol 2005;185(1):64–71.

21. Ginat DT, Saad W, Davies M, et al. Bowel displacement for CT-guided tumor radiofrequency ablation: techniques and anatomic considerations. J Endourol 2009;23(8):1259–64.

22. Cantwell CP, Wah TM, Gervais DA, et al. Protecting the ureter during radiofrequency ablation of renal cell cancer: a pilot study of retrograde pyeloperfusion with cooled dextrose 5% in water. J Vasc Interv Radiol 2008;19(7):1034–40.

23. Gervais DA, Arellano RS, McGovern FJ, et al. Radiofrequency ablation of renal cell carcinoma: part 2. Lessons learned with ablation of 100 tumors. AJR Am J Roentgenol 2005;185(1):72–80.

24. Hoffmann NE, Bischof JC. The cryobiology of cryosurgical injury. Urology 2002;60(2 Suppl 1):40–9.

25. Lovelock JE. The haemolysis of human red blood-cells by freezing and thawing. Biochim Biophys Acta 1953;10(3):414–26.

26. Daum PS, Bowers WD Jr, Tejada J, et al. Vascular casts demonstrate microcirculatory insufficiency in acute frostbite. Cryobiology 1987;24(1):65–73.

27. Hoffmann NE, Bischof JC. Cryosurgery of normal and tumor tissue in the dorsal skin flap chamber: part II–injury response. J Biomech Eng 2001;123(4):310–6.

28. Finelli A, Rewcastle JC, Jewett MA. Cryotherapy and radiofrequency ablation: pathophysiologic basis and laboratory studies. Curr Opin Urol 2003;13(3): 187–91.

29. Matin SF, Sharma P, Gill IS, et al. Immunological response to renal cryoablation in an in vivo orthotopic renal cell carcinoma murine model. J Urol 2010;183(1):333–8.

30. Sidana A, Chowdhury WH, Fuchs EJ, et al. Cryoimmunotherapy in urologic oncology. Urology 2010;75(5):1009–14.

31. Permpongkosol S, Nielsen ME, Solomon SB. Percutaneous renal cryoablation. Urology 2006;68(Suppl 1):19–25.

32. Woolley ML, Schulsinger DA, Durand DB, et al. Effect of freezing parameters (freeze cycle and thaw process) on tissue destruction following renal cryoablation. J Endourol 2002;16(7):519–22.

33. Aron M, Gill IS. Minimally invasive nephron-sparing surgery (MINSS) for renal tumours. Part II: probe ablative therapy. Eur Urol 2007;51(2):348–57.

34. Matin SF, Ahrar K, Cadeddu JA, et al. Residual and recurrent disease following renal energy ablative therapy: a multi-institutional study. J Urol 2006;176(5): 1973–7.

35. Matsumoto ED, Watumull L, Johnson DB, et al. The radiographic evolution of radio frequency ablated renal tumors. J Urol 2004;172(1):45–8.

36. Weight CJ, Kaouk JH, Hegarty NJ, et al. Correlation of radiographic imaging and histopathology following cryoablation and radio frequency ablation for renal tumors. J Urol 2008;179(4):1277–81 [discussion: 1281–3].

37. Matin SF. Determining failure after renal ablative therapy for renal cell carcinoma: false-negative and false-positive imaging findings. Urology 2010;75(6):1254–7.

38. Lucas SM, Stern JM, Adibi M, et al. Renal function outcomes in patients treated for renal masses smaller than 4 cm by ablative and extirpative techniques. J Urol 2008;179(1):75–9 [discussion: 79–80].

39. Raman JD, Raj GV, Lucas SM, et al. Renal functional outcomes for tumours in a solitary kidney managed by ablative or extirpative techniques. BJU Int 2010; 105(4):496–500.

40. Weisbrod AJ, Atwell TD, Frank I, et al. Percutaneous cryoablation of masses in a solitary kidney. AJR Am J Roentgenol 2010;194(6):1620–5.

41. Ahrar K, Matin S, Wood CG, et al. Percutaneous radiofrequency ablation of renal tumors: technique, complications, and outcomes. J Vasc Interv Radiol 2005; 16(5):679–88.

42. Mahnken AH, Rohde D, Brkovic D, et al. Percutaneous radiofrequency ablation of renal cell carcinoma: preliminary results. Acta Radiol 2005;46(2):208–14.

43. Matsumoto ED, Johnson DB, Ogan K, et al. Short-term efficacy of temperature-based radiofrequency ablation of small renal tumors. Urology 2005;65(5):877–81.

44. Arzola J, Baughman SM, Hernandez J, et al. Computed tomography-guided, resistance-based, percutaneous radiofrequency ablation of renal malignancies under conscious sedation at two years of follow-up. Urology 2006;68(5):983–7.

45. Park S, Anderson JK, Matsumoto ED, et al. Radiofrequency ablation of renal tumors: intermediate-term results. J Endourol 2006;20(8):569–73.

46. Carey RI, Leveillee RJ. First prize: direct real-time temperature monitoring for laparoscopic and CT-guided radiofrequency ablation of renal tumors between 3 and 5 cm. J Endourol 2007;21(8):807–13.

47. Stern JM, Svatek R, Park S, et al. Intermediate comparison of partial nephrectomy and radiofrequency ablation for clinical T1a renal tumours. BJU Int 2007;100(2): 287–90.
48. Breen DJ, Rutherford EE, Stedman B, et al. Management of renal tumors by image-guided radiofrequency ablation: experience in 105 tumors. Cardiovasc Intervent Radiol 2007;30(5):936–42.
49. Levinson AW, Su LM, Agarwal D, et al. Long-term oncological and overall outcomes of percutaneous radio frequency ablation in high risk surgical patients with a solitary small renal mass. J Urol 2008;180(2):499–504 [discussion: 504].
50. Hoffmann RT, Jakobs TF, Kubisch CH, et al. Renal cell carcinoma in patients with a solitary kidney after nephrectomy treated with radiofrequency ablation: mid term results. Eur J Radiol 2010;73(3):652–6.
51. del Cura JL, Zabala R, Iriarte JI, et al. Treatment of renal tumors by percutaneous ultrasound-guided radiofrequency ablation using a multitined electrode: effectiveness and complications. Eur Urol 2010;57(3):459–65.
52. Gill IS, Remer EM, Hasan WA, et al. Renal cryoablation: outcome at 3 years. J Urol 2005;173(6):1903–7.
53. Silverman SG, Tuncali K, vanSonnenberg E, et al. Renal tumors: MR imaging-guided percutaneous cryotherapy–initial experience in 23 patients. Radiology 2005;236(2):716–24.
54. Davol PE, Fulmer BR, Rukstalis DB. Long-term results of cryoablation for renal cancer and complex renal masses. Urology 2006;68(Suppl 1):2–6.
55. Gupta A, Allaf ME, Kavoussi LR, et al. Computerized tomography guided percutaneous renal cryoablation with the patient under conscious sedation: initial clinical experience. J Urol 2006;175(2):447–52 [discussion: 452–3].
56. Schwartz BF, Rewcastle JC, Powell T, et al. Cryoablation of small peripheral renal masses: a retrospective analysis. Urology 2006;68(Suppl 1):14–8.
57. Miki K, Shimomura T, Yamada H, et al. Percutaneous cryoablation of renal cell carcinoma guided by horizontal open magnetic resonance imaging. Int J Urol 2006;13(7):880–4.
58. Weld KJ, Figenshau RS, Venkatesh R, et al. Laparoscopic cryoablation for small renal masses: three-year follow-up. Urology 2007;69(3):448–51.
59. Wyler SF, Sulser T, Ruszat R, et al. Intermediate-term results of retroperitoneoscopy-assisted cryotherapy for small renal tumours using multiple ultrathin cryoprobes. Eur Urol 2007;51(4):971–9.
60. Bandi G, Wen CC, Hedican SP, et al. Cryoablation of small renal masses: assessment of the outcome at one institution. BJU Int 2007;100(4):798–801.
61. Atwell TD, Farrell MA, Callstrom MR, et al. Percutaneous cryoablation of 40 solid renal tumors with US guidance and CT monitoring: initial experience. Radiology 2007;243(1):276–83.
62. Atwell TD, Farrell MA, Leibovich BC, et al. Percutaneous renal cryoablation: experience treating 115 tumors. J Urol 2008;179(6):2136–40 [discussion: 2140–1].
63. Finley DS, Beck S, Box G, et al. Percutaneous and laparoscopic cryoablation of small renal masses. J Urol 2008;180(2):492–8 [discussion: 498].
64. Malcolm JB, Berry TT, Williams MB, et al. Single center experience with percutaneous and laparoscopic cryoablation of small renal masses. J Endourol 2009; 23(6):907–11.
65. Schmit GD, Atwell TD, Callstrom MR, et al. Percutaneous cryoablation of renal masses > or =3 cm: efficacy and safety in treatment of 108 patients. J Endourol 2010;24(8):1255–62.

66. Aron M, Kamoi K, Remer E, et al. Laparoscopic renal cryoablation: 8-year, single surgeon outcomes. J Urol 2010;183(3):889–95.
67. Chawla SN, Crispen PL, Hanlon AL, et al. The natural history of observed enhancing renal masses: meta-analysis and review of the world literature. J Urol 2006;175(2):425–31.
68. Campbell SC, Novick AC, Belldegrun A, et al. Guideline for management of the clinical T1 renal mass. J Urol 2009;182(4):1271–9.
69. Tsivian M, Lyne JC, Mayes JM, et al. Tumor size and endophytic growth pattern affect recurrence rates after laparoscopic renal cryoablation. Urology 2010;75(2): 307–10.
70. Yoost TR, Clarke HS, Savage SJ. Laparoscopic cryoablation of renal masses: which lesions fail? Urology 2010;75(2):311–4.
71. Johnson DB, Solomon SB, Su LM, et al. Defining the complications of cryoablation and radio frequency ablation of small renal tumors: a multi-institutional review. J Urol 2004;172(3):874–7.
72. Bhayani SB, Allaf ME, Su LM, et al. Neuromuscular complications after percutaneous radiofrequency ablation of renal tumors. Urology 2005;65(3):592.
73. Weizer AZ, Raj GV, O'Connell M, et al. Complications after percutaneous radiofrequency ablation of renal tumors. Urology 2005;66(6):1176–80.
74. Nguyen CT, Lane BR, Kaouk JH, et al. Surgical salvage of renal cell carcinoma recurrence after thermal ablative therapy. J Urol 2008;180(1):104–9 [discussion: 109].
75. Kowalczyk KJ, Hooper HB, Linehan WM, et al. Partial nephrectomy after previous radio frequency ablation: the National Cancer Institute experience. J Urol 2009; 182(5):2158–63.

Ablation of Bone Metastases

Javier Nazario, MD[a,b], Alda L. Tam, MD, FRCPC, MBA[a,*]

KEYWORDS
- Percutaneous ablation • Radiofrequency ablation
- Cryoablation • Bone metastases • Pain palliation

Osseous metastases are a common problem for patients with cancer; up to 85% of patients with breast, prostate, and lung cancer have evidence of bone metastases at the time of death.[1] Although most bone metastases are asymptomatic, osseous metastases are a common cause of cancer-related pain and can be quite debilitating, affecting patients' quality of life, performance status, and mood.[2–4]

A multidisciplinary team approach with collaborative efforts between medical oncologists, radiation oncologists, surgical oncologists, and interventional radiologists is often necessary to determine optimal therapy as various treatment modalities are available for the management of osseous metastases. Treatments for painful bone metastases are usually palliative. Surgery is generally reserved for stabilization purposes and has a limited role in the palliation of painful bone metastases without pathologic fracture.[5,6] Systemic therapies (chemotherapy, hormonal therapy, radiopharmaceuticals, and bisphosphonates) have specific yet limited usefulness because painful osseous metastatic disease is usually refractory to standard chemotherapy and hormonal therapy.[6] Analgesics (opioids and nonsteroidal antiinflammatory drugs) remain a cornerstone treatment for many patients with painful bone metastases. However, to achieve adequate levels of pain control, higher doses of these medications are frequently required and can lead to significant side effects, including constipation and over sedation.[7]

External beam radiation therapy (XRT) is the current standard of care for the palliation of patients with cancer with painful bone metastases. However, published reports in the literature indicate that many patients do not achieve optimal relief, with up to

There was no grant support.
The authors have nothing to disclose.
[a] Vascular and Interventional Radiology, The University of Texas, MD Anderson Cancer Center, Houston, TX, USA
[b] Interventional Radiology Department, Hospital HIMA-San Pablo, PO Box 236, Bayamón, PR 00960-6036, USA
* Corresponding author. Department of Diagnostic Radiology, Section of Interventional Radiology, The University of Texas, MD Anderson Cancer Center, PO Box 301402, Houston, TX 77230-1402.
E-mail address: alda.tam@mdanderson.org

30% of patients experiencing inadequate analgesia following XRT.[3,8,9] Moreover, the onset of pain relief is often delayed for up to 4 to 12 weeks following therapy and the durability of pain relief can be short lived with many patients experiencing recurrent pain within months of XRT therapy.[9,10] Unfortunately, previously irradiated sites are often not eligible for further XRT because of the limitations of normal tissue tolerance.[7]

Image-guided percutaneous ablation techniques have several advantages that address the limitations of XRT and have become an important palliative treatment option in patients with painful bone metastases. The most commonly used methods are radiofrequency ablation (RFA) and cryoablation. The purpose of this article is to summarize the techniques for image-guided ablation of bone metastases and to review the literature on its use in the palliation of bone pain.

PATIENT SELECTION AND PREPROCEDURE MANAGEMENT

In the palliative setting, ablative techniques are indicated for patients with painful osteolytic bone metastases who are not suitable candidates for or have failed other standard forms of therapy. Although there is no limit to the size of the tumor that can be treated, patients' pain must be limited, from 1 or 2 sites of metastatic disease in bone, and should rate greater than or equal to 4 on a pain scale of 0 to 10. Contra-indications include tumors that are in direct contact with hollow viscera or neural elements. In general, the edge of the ablation zone should be at least 1 cm away from the spinal cord, major motor nerves, brain, artery of Adamkiewicz, bowel, or bladder. Lesions in weight-bearing bones should be treated only if there is no risk of an impending fracture. Patients with recurrent tumors at sites that have been surgically stabilized with metallic hardware are not candidates for RFA but may be eligible for cryoablation. Hypervascular bone metastases larger than 3 or 4 cm may be more suit-able for cryoablation because perfusion-mediated tissue cooling may prevent effec-tive RFA ablation. However, preablation arterial embolization of these large, hypervascular tumors can be performed to address this problem and to potentiate the effects of RFA[4,11] (**Fig. 1** A, B, C, D, E). Finally, treatment of osteoblastic lesions is infrequently performed because of the often difficult access through sclerotic bone and poor RFA energy deposition in these lesions.[3]

Before any image-guided intervention, adequate imaging of the affected site must be obtained for procedure planning. In particular, cross-sectional imaging with computed tomography (CT) or MRI is necessary to assess the extent of disease and the proximity of the lesion to vital structures.[12] Patients should be examined before the procedure to determine the location and severity of the pain. Validated pain scales, such as the Brief Pain Inventory and the Memorial Pain Assessment Card (MPAC), are useful tools for scoring pain severity and provide baseline data for outcome analysis. Lastly, patients' opioid analgesic use should be inventoried and translated to a morphine-equivalent dose for future comparison.[11]

The platelet count should be greater than 75,000/μL and coagulopathies should be corrected. Anticoagulation medications, such as aspirin, antiplatelet medications, low molecular weight heparin preparations and warfarin, should be discontinued before the procedure.

METHODS OF ABLATION

Several image-guided thermal ablation technologies have been developed and used in the ablation of painful bone metastases, including RFA, cryoablation, microwave ablation, laser interstitial thermal therapy, plasma-mediated RF (coablation), and focused ultrasound therapy[6,13–15]; however, this review focuses on the most studied

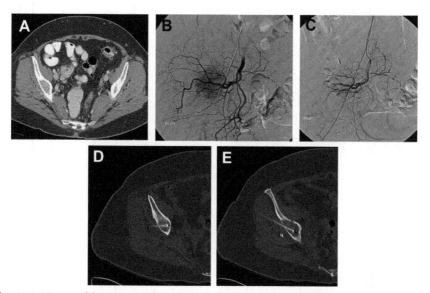

Fig. 1. A 70-year-old woman with a history of metastatic renal cell carcinoma and solitary right iliac bone metastasis. The patient was having increasing right hip pain. (*A*) Axial, contrast-enhanced CT image demonstrates a hypervascular, lytic right iliac bone lesion, measuring approximately 3.5 cm in dimension. Because of the lesion's size and hypervascularity, perfusion-mediated tissue cooling during RFA ablation was a concern and pre-RFA embolization was planned. (*B*) Digital subtraction angiography from the right internal iliac artery demonstrates significant hypervascularity of the right iliac mass, supplied by branches of the posterior division of the right internal iliac artery. Multiple branches were superselectively embolized using a coaxial microcatheter and 300- to 500-μm tris-acryl microspheres. (*C*) Post-embolization angiography from the right internal iliac artery demonstrates significant reduction in the hypervascularity in the right iliac mass. (*D, E*) The patient returned the following day to undergo RFA of the right iliac lesion. Two 15-cm ValleyLab Cool Tip RFA probes, with 2-cm active tips, were inserted to cover the cephalad (*D*) and caudal (*E*) aspects of the lesion. Multiple overlapping ablations were performed at each level. The duration of each ablation was 6 minutes. Postablation temperatures at all sites measured greater than 70°C.

and most commonly used ablation methods, which are RFA and cryoablation. Although the exact mechanism of pain relief following ablation is unclear, it is likely multifactorial and several theories have been put forth. RFA and cryoablation may contribute to relief of tumor-related bone pain by: (1) destroying local sensory nerves supplying the periosteum thereby inhibiting pain transmission, (2) reducing tumor volume thus decreasing the stimulation of sensory nerve fibers, (3) destroying cytokine-producing tumor cells, and (4) inhibiting osteoclast activity.[16]

A summary of the reported studies regarding the use of thermal ablative techniques in the palliative treatment of pain related to osseous metastatic disease is provided in **Table 1**. Generally, most studies demonstrate that percutaneous ablative techniques used in this setting are safe and achieve durable palliation in this cohort of patients with limited life expectancy and pain refractory to standard therapies. Nevertheless, extrapolation of these results is limited because of the different parameters used to objectively assess patients' pain, the heterogeneity of lesions treated (location, pathology, and size), different ablative techniques used (RFA vs cryoablation), and the length of follow-up. Reporting standards and guidelines should be followed to adequately compare trials in the future.[17]

Table 1
Summary of studies using percutaneous ablation techniques for the palliation of pain related to bone metastases

Author	N	Ablation Method	Prior Treatment	Tumor Size (mean or range)	Pain Assessment Scale	Pretreatment Pain Score Baseline	Pretreatment Pain Score Worst	Posttreatment Pain Score Baseline	Posttreatment Pain Score Worst	P-Value	Study Follow-Up Period	Additional Comments
Dupuy et al 2010[4]	55	RFA	NR	5.2 cm	mMPAC	54.4	91.0	14.2	NR	0.02	3 months	—
Carrafiello et al 2009[19]	10	RFA/plasma mediated RF ± cementoplasty	100%	1.4–8.8 cm	VAS	8.0	NR	2.0	NR	<0.001	3 months	MED decreased from 80–100 to 30–40 at 3 months (P < .001)
Tuncali et al 2007[30]	10	Cryoablation	NR	5.2 cm	NR	NR	NR	NR	NR	NR	1–44 weeks (mean 8.9)	17 of 19 pts had pain palliation (6 of 17 complete, 11of 17 partial)
Callstrom et al 2005[6]	14	Cryoablation	100%	4.3 cm (1.0–11.0 cm)	BPI, VAS	4.5	6.7	2.0	3.4	0.003	8 weeks	No statistically significant change in MED
Poggi et al 2003[21]	5	RFA	100%	3.0 to 8.0 cm	VAS	NR	NR	NR	NR	NR	NR	4 of 5 pts had pain palliation (1 pt free up to 88 weeks)
Goetz et al 2002[23]	43	RFA	77%	6.3 cm	BPI-sf	5.8	7.9	1.2	1.4	0.005	24 weeks	No statistically significant change in MED
Callstrom et al 2002[16]	12	RFA	100%	4.9 cm (1.3–10.8 cm)	BPI, VAS	6.5	8.0	1.4	2.4	<0.04	1–24 weeks (mean 8)	8 of 10 pts reduced analgesic medication post-RFA
Gronemeyer et al 2001[22]	10	RFA	100%	1.5 to 9.0 cm	VAS	59.5	NR	26.0	NR	NR	2–11 months	—

Abbreviations: BPI, Brief Pain Inventory; BPI-sf, Brief Pain Inventory short form; MED, morphine equivalent dose; mMPAC, modified Memorial Pain Assessment Card; NR, not reported; pts, patients; RF/RFA, radiofrequency ablation; VAS, visual analog scale.

RADIOFREQUENCY ABLATION

Radiofrequency ablation uses a high-frequency alternating current (375–500 kHz) to deposit thermal energy (heat) into tissue, resulting in ionic agitation, frictional heating, and ultimately coagulative necrosis. Sources of heat loss, such as the proximity of large blood vessels, can limit the volume of ablation. Temperatures must be maintained between 60° to 100°C to ensure irreversible cell damage.[18] Three RFA systems are commercially available in the United States and are manufactured by Boston Scientific (BOS; Natick, MA, USA), RITA (Angiodynamics Inc, Queensbury, NY, USA), and Valleylab (VL; Boulder, CO, USA). RFA electrodes range from 14 to 17 gauge. They also vary in shape with some having an expandable tine design and others are simply straight.

In addition to many retrospective series,[16,19–23] 2 prospective trials[4,24] have demonstrated the efficacy of using percutaneous image-guided RFA for pain palliation of bone metastases (see **Table 1**). In 2002, Goetz and colleagues[24] published the results of a multicenter, prospective trial involving the RFA treatment of 43 subjects with severe bone pain. Significant pain relief, defined as at least a 2-point drop in worst pain score, was achieved in 41 of 43 subjects (95%) following RFA. In addition, the onset of pain relief was rapid as 41% (17 of 41 subjects) achieved at least a 2-point drop in worst or average pain by the first week and 59% (24 of 41 subjects) did so by the fourth week. The results were significant because of the degree of pain relief achieved and because this degree of relief was achieved in a subject population traditionally refractory to conventional treatment.[24]

Most recently, a multicenter, single-arm prospective American College of Radiology Imaging Network trial was completed.[4] A total of 55 subjects underwent RFA for palliative treatment of intractable pain from a single-bone metastases that measured greater than 50 on a pain scale of 1 to 100. Pain assessment was performed before and after RFA using a modified MPAC. The authors found that RFA reduced pain for all MPAC pain assessment measures. The average increase in pain relief was 26.3 ($P<.0001$) and 16.38 ($P = .02$) at 1-month and 3-month follow-up, respectively. The average decrease in pain intensity was 26.9 ($P<.0001$) and 14.2 ($P = .02$) at 1-month and 3-month follow-up, respectively. The average increase in mood was 19.9 ($P<.0001$) and 14.9 ($P = .005$) at 1-month and 3-month follow-up, respectively. Grade 3 toxicities occurred in 3 subjects (5%) and consisted of pain from RFA, neuropathic pain, and foot drop. The study demonstrated that RFA for bone metastases could be safely performed and provides durable palliation for pain related to bone metastases in a cooperative group setting. The authors suggest that further research in the form of a randomized controlled trial is warranted to further evaluate this treatment option.[4]

CRYOABLATION

Cryoablation has a long history of successful treatment of neoplasms in the prostate, kidney, liver, and uterus.[6] The development of lower-profile, insulated cryoprobes that use room temperature argon gas have made this technology suitable for image-guided percutaneous ablation. The delivery of argon gas through a segmentally insulated probe, with rapid expansion of the gas, results in rapid cooling (Thompson-Joule effect). Temperatures can reach -100°C within seconds. The outer edge of the ice ball corresponds to 0°C and cell death occurs at temperatures of -20°C and below, which is about 3-mm deep to the ice ball margin.[25,26] There are 3 proposed mechanisms of cryoinjury.[27] First, the formation of ice crystals within the cell leads to direct cellular injury with protein denaturation and membrane disruption. Second, freezing results in the coagulation of blood and stasis in the microcirculation, which leads to ischemia and subsequent necrosis. Finally, some authors have suggested that cryoablation may sensitize the immune system and induce apoptotic cell death. The size of the ice ball that is generated varies depending on the length of the uninsulated tip, the volume of gas passing through the probe, and the freezing time.[3] The thawing process is achieved by the installation of helium gas into the cryoprobe. Two cryoablation systems are commercially available in the United States and are manufactured by Endocare, Inc (HealthTronics, Inc, Austin, TX, USA) and Galil Medical (Arden Hills, MN, USA). Cryoablation probes have diameters of 12 mm, 17 mm, and 24 mm (17, 11, and 13 gauge, respectively). A single cryoprobe usually creates an oblong ice ball that is 3.5 cm in diameter.

A cryoablation treatment consists of 10 minutes of freezing followed by 5 minutes of thawing and a second 10 minutes of freezing. Shorter or longer freezing or thawing times are used depending on the adequacy of coverage of the lesion and the proximity of adjacent critical structures. Cryoablation has several advantages over RFA. Ice is a natural anesthetic and patients have reported decreased pain during and following the procedure. Ice is visible by imaging and this allows for the ablation margin to be reliably defined and increases the likelihood that a lesion will be completely ablated. Ice propagation is predictable and reproducible and gives the operator improved control during the ablation.[3] Lastly, cryoablation may be more advantageous in the treatment of sclerotic metastases because ice can penetrate deeply into bone as opposed to RFA, which penetrates poorly into bone.[28]

Callstrom and colleagues[29] have reported interim results on an ongoing prospective clinical trial in which 14 subjects were treated with image-guided percutaneous cryoablation for painful bone metastases and demonstrated significant reductions in pain (see **Table 1**). Treated lesion sizes ranged from 1.0 to 11.0 cm. The number of cryoprobes used for the ablation procedure ranged from 1 to 7. The total cryoablation procedure time ranged from 83 to 280 minutes. During the follow-up period of 24 weeks, 12 of 14 subjects (86%) reported at least a 3-point drop in worst pain during the first 24-hour period. The subjects also reported an improved quality of life following cryoablation. No major complications were reported. The subject characteristics and response to therapy were similar to subjects treated in the 2002 multicenter RFA trial.[24] Although there are no studies directly comparing RFA and cryoablation for the palliation of pain caused by bone metastases, the reported pain scores following cryoablation are statistically similar to the pain scores reported after RFA treatment.

More recently, Tuncali and colleagues[30] reported on the safety and feasibility of percutaneous MRI-guided cryotherapy in the care of subjects with refractory or painful metastatic lesions of soft tissue and bone adjacent to or encasing critical structures, such as the bowel, bladder, or major blood vessels. Palliation was achieved in 17 of 19 subjects (89%) treated for pain with 6 subjects experiencing complete pain relief. Complications (n = 6) included 2 subjects with transient lower extremity numbness, 2 subjects with both urinary retention and transient lower extremity paresthesia, 1 subject with chronic vaginal discharge, and 1 subject who fractured their femoral neck at the ablation site 6 weeks following treatment. The authors conclude that MRI-guided cryoablation was safe when ablating tumors adjacent to critical structures.

TECHNICAL CONSIDERATIONS

Image-guided percutaneous ablation of bone metastases can be performed under conscious sedation, regional anesthesia, or general anesthesia. CT is the most common form of imaging guidance for percutaneous ablation although both MRI and ultrasound can be used to guide probe placement. For osteolytic lesions where the cortical bone has been disrupted, the RFA electrodes or cryoprobes can be placed directly into the lesion. When the cortical bone is intact, a bone biopsy needle (11 or 13 gauge) or a bone drill may have to be used to create an access to the lesion to allow for RFA electrode or cryoprobe placement.

The size of the RFA ablation that can be generated is dependent on the probe configuration that is being used. Often, multiple, overlapping RFA ablations will be required to treat larger tumors. Although there is no set algorithm, typically ablations of 5 to 10 minutes are performed at the target temperature of 100°C or until tissue impedance limits the delivery of additional energy. Postablation temperatures should measure more than 60°C (**Fig. 2** A, B, C, D).

One of the advantages of cryoablation is the ability to use multiple (up to 25) cryoprobes simultaneously, which allows for the formation of large ice balls (>8 cm in diameter).[6] Multiple cryoprobes can also be placed in a manner that creates ice balls of various geometric configurations, which can be designed to cover the entire tumor with one ablation. Because of the oblong shape of the ice ball, cryoprobes are usually

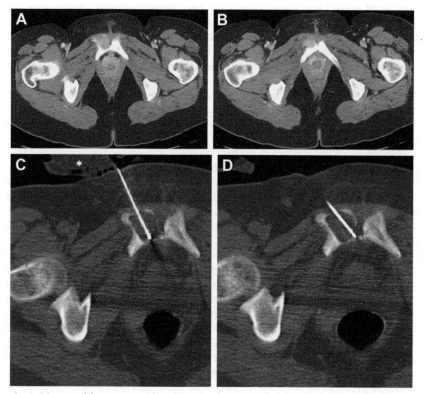

Fig. 2. A 36-year-old woman with a history of metastatic alveolar soft part sarcoma and right-sided pelvic pain that was not well controlled on oral analgesic medications. (*A, B*) Axial, contrast-enhanced CT images demonstrate a 2.5 × 1.7-cm lytic lesion of the right superior pubic ramus with an associated enhancing soft-tissue component. (*C, D*) RFA of the right pubic ramus lesion was performed for pain palliation. A ValleyLab Cool Tip RFA probe with a 2-cm active tip was used to ablate the lesion along its long axis. Multiple overlapping ablations were performed to target the lateral (*C*) and medial (*D*) margins of the lesion. An ice pack (*) was placed on the skin surface (*C*) to prevent thermal injury to the overlying skin.

placed in parallel to the long axis of the tumor. When multiple cryoprobes are used, they are usually placed in parallel 2 cm apart from each other with the peripheral probes placed 1 cm from the tumor margin. During the cryoablation procedure, limited noncontrast CT imaging is performed as often as every 2 minutes throughout the freezing portions of the cycle to monitor the growth of the ice ball. Following completion of the final freeze of the cryoablation, the cryoprobes are warmed with active thawing with helium and then withdrawn.

One of the disadvantages of cryoablation as compared with RFA is that it takes on average 30- to 60-minutes longer than a RFA procedure.[3] Several reasons contribute to this increased procedure time: the actual cryoablation treatment takes about 25 to 30 minutes compared with 5 to 10 minutes for an RFA treatment; it takes longer to place the cryoprobes; and additional time can be spent maximizing the size of the ice ball, so more than one freeze-thaw-freeze cycle may be performed.[29] Furthermore, because of the ability to design specific geometric shapes, more cryoprobes are often used as compared with RFA and this can make cryoablation more expensive than RFA.

The goal for pain palliation cases is complete ablation of the bone–soft-tissue interface (**Fig. 3** A, B, C, D). For certain patients with slow-growing, oligometastatic disease, local control may be achieved with percutaneous ablation techniques if the ablation margin can be extended sufficiently beyond the confines of the tumor (**Fig. 4** A, B, C, D, E, F). A fundamental distinction between RFA and cryoablation is that the ablation margin is not visible with RFA. Some authors have suggested that this inability to see the ablation zone may lead to incomplete tumor ablation, particularly at the margins close to critical structures.[6]

When the lesion to be ablated is in close proximity to critical structures, various techniques can be used to minimize the potential for collateral damage to normal tissue. Placement of a thermocouple next to a critical structure can be used to provide real-time temperature monitoring during an ablation procedure (**Fig. 5** A, B, C, D, E). The temperature of the nontarget, normal structure should not reach greater than or equal to 45°C in RFA cases or less than or equal to 8°C in cryoablation cases.[31,32] Tissue displacement techniques include hydrodissection with sterile water (usually dextrose 5% in water [D5W]) in RFA and saline in cryoablation, and the use of balloons to push critical structures away from the ablation margin. Furthermore, the injection of CO_2 gas to insulate critical structures, such as the spinal cord and nerves, has also been reported[31] (see **Fig. 5**).

Currently, there has been increasing interest in the use of ablation followed by percutaneous cementoplasty in the treatment of bone metastases at risk for fracture in axial-loading locations, such as the vertebral body or the periacetabular region[3,32–35] (see **Fig. 5**). It is thought that the coagulative necrosis seen after RFA promotes a more even distribution of the cement, which is injected to provide stabilization and reduce the risk of subsequent fracture.[23,36] RFA followed by cementoplasty can be completed in one procedural setting; however, cryoablation followed by cementoplasty usually requires that the procedures be performed on successive days because it can take up to 1 hour for the ice ball to thaw completely.[3] Patients who have undergone these combination procedures have also experienced significant pain relief.[32–35]

COMPLICATIONS

Complications related to percutaneous ablation of bone lesions are rare but include skin burns, frostbite, hemorrhage, infection, and fracture. Depending on the region treated, neurologic adverse events can be seen, including incomplete hemiplegia, radiculopathy, and transient bowel and bladder incontinence.[16,24,32]

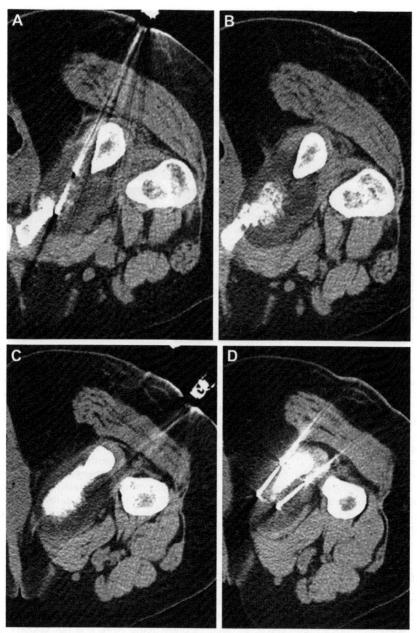

Fig. 3. A 35-year-old woman with metastatic colorectal cancer and mixed osteolytic/osteo-blastic metastasis of the left pubic ramus. The patient had undergone palliative radiation to the pelvis but continued to have persistent, severe, left pelvic pain. Cryoablation was per-formed for pain palliation and complete ablation of the bone soft-tissue interface was the goal. (*A, B, C, D*) A total of 5 24-mm cryoprobes (Endocare, Inc [HealthTronics, Inc, Austin, TX, USA]) were placed to encompass the lesion. The oblong-shaped ice ball is identified as the low-density area surrounding the partially sclerotic pubic bone.

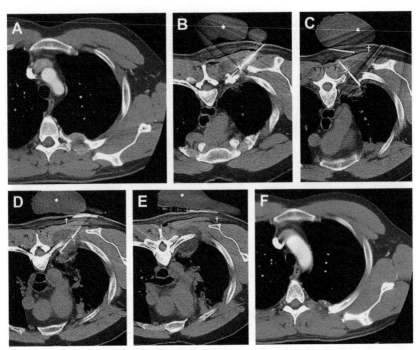

Fig. 4. A 47-year-old man with a history of renal cell carcinoma and a solitary rib metastasis. Cryoablation was requested for local control of disease. (*A*) Axial, contrast-enhanced CT image demonstrates a 3.5-cm hypervascular metastasis involving the posterior left fourth rib. One 17-mm cryoprobe (*B*) and 2 24-mm cryoprobes (*C, D*) (Endocare, Inc [HealthTronics, Inc, Austin, TX, USA]) were placed in a crisscross fashion to span the lesion. Saline was injected subcutaneously (†) through an 18-gauge needle to create a (salinoma), displacing the skin surface from the outer edge of the ice ball. A warm saline compress (*) was also placed on the skin surface to decrease the risk of thermal injury to the skin. The resulting hypodense ice ball (*B, C, D, E*) completely covers the lytic lesion with a sufficient margin to ensure adequate ablation for local control. Crossing the probes changed the configuration of the resulting ice ball. Instead of the oblong shape normally generated from a single probe, this configuration created a cube-shaped ice ball with a maximum dimension of 5.5 cm. (*F*) Axial, contrast-enhanced CT image approximately 1 year following cryoablation demonstrates the lesion in the left fourth rib is smaller in size and nonenhancing.

POSTPROCEDURE MANAGEMENT AND FOLLOW-UP

Although these procedures can be performed on an outpatient basis, patients with moderate to severe pain are often observed in the hospital overnight and their pain managed with opioid analgesics. In patients undergoing RFA, it is not uncommon for the pain to become more severe in the immediate postprocedure period. The use of patient-controlled analgesia, regional anesthetic blocks, or epidural anesthesia can be helpful for patients undergoing RFA in the immediate postprocedure period. In contrast, patients undergoing cryoablation do not typically experience increased pain in the postprocedure period. For all patients undergoing ablation, it is expected that the pain will return to at least baseline after the first day. Once patients' pain can be controlled with oral pain medication, they can be discharged. Significant decreases in pain intensity can be expected within 1 month of the procedure.

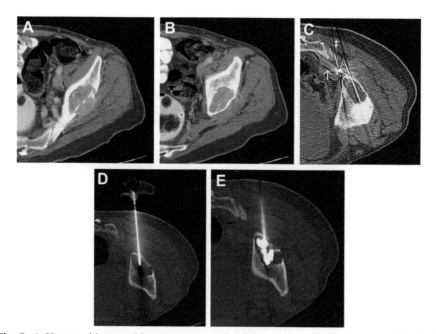

Fig. 5. A 63-year-old man with metastatic renal cell carcinoma. The patient complained of excruciating left hip pain and cryoablation was requested for pain palliation. (*A, B*) Axial, contrast-enhanced images demonstrate a lytic lesion involving the left iliac bone, extending down into the acetabulum. Two 24-mm cryoprobes (Endocare, Inc [HealthTronics, Inc, Austin, TX, USA]) were placed within the iliac bone, targeting the bone soft-tissue interface (not shown). (*C*) A 17-mm cryoprobe (Endocare, Inc [HealthTronics, Inc, Austin, TX, USA]) was placed within the acetabular portion of the lesion. Because of the proximity of the posterior border of the lesion to the sciatic notch, other protective techniques, in addition to routine CT monitoring of the ice ball progression, were used to monitor for potential injury to the left sciatic nerve. Sural nerve stimulation was performed throughout the procedure to assess the integrity of the sciatic nerve. A 21-gauge needle was used to inject CO_2 gas around the left sciatic nerve and this can be seen as air tracking along the fascial planes as denoted by the ↑ in (*C*). A 17-gauge thermocouple (Endocare, Inc [HealthTronics, Inc, Austin, TX, USA]) marked as ‡ in (*C*) was placed adjacent to the left sciatic nerve, which provided real-time monitoring of the temperature near the nerve during cryoablation. (*D, E*) As the lesion involved the acetabulum, cryoablation was followed by cementoplasty the next day to reduce the potential risk for fracture. Two 13-gauge vertebroplasty needles (Cook Inc, Bloomington, IN, USA) were placed and a total of 5 mL of polymethylmethacrylate was injected into the acetabular roof under CT guidance.

Unlike ablation in solid organs, such as lung, liver, and kidney, there is no defined follow-up imaging algorithm. For patients with oligometastatic disease where local control is the goal, regular, staging examinations should be used to determine if repeat ablation is necessary. In palliation cases, the clinical assessment of benefit is more meaningful and pain severity and opioid usage should be monitored.

SUMMARY

Cancer pain is a significant health issue. Considering the reduced life expectancy in patients with advanced neoplasm, an ideal procedure for the palliation of bone pain should provide durable relief in a timely manner, improve patients' quality of life, decrease hospitalizations, and be well tolerated.[12] In some aspects, percutaneous ablation technologies offer distinct advantages over XRT: cell death is immediate, the onset of pain relief is more rapid, the bone can be stabilized with cement injection, and the minimally invasive procedure can be repeated at the same site should the tumor recur.[12,37] RFA and cryoablation have been shown to be precise and safe treatments in the palliation of painful bone metastases refractory to standard therapies and should be incorporated into the treatment algorithm of managing osseous metastatic disease.

REFERENCES

1. Nielsen OS, Munro AJ, Tannock IF. Bone metastases: pathophysiology and management policy. J Clin Oncol 1991;9:509–24.
2. Twycross R, Harcourt J, Bergl S. A survey of pain in patients with advanced cancer. J Pain Symptom Manage 1996;12:273–82.
3. Callstrom MR, Charboneau JW. Image-guided palliation of painful metastases using percutaneous ablation. Tech Vasc Interv Radiol 2007;10(2):120–31.
4. Dupuy DE, Liu D, Hartfell D, et al. Percutaneous radiofrequency ablation of painful osseous metastases: a multicenter American College of Radiology Imaging Network trial. Cancer 2010;116:989–97.
5. Aboulafia AJ, Levine AM, Schmidt D, et al. Surgical therapy of bone metastases. Semin Oncol 2007;34(3):206–14.
6. Callstrom MR, Kurup AN. Percutaneous ablation for bone and soft tissue metastases: why cryoablation? Skeletal Radiol 2009;38:835–9.
7. Callstrom MR, Charboneau JW. Percutaneous ablation: safe, effective treatment of bone tumors. Oncology 2005;19(11):22–6.
8. Agarawal JP, Swangsilpa T, van der Linden Y, et al. The role of external beam radiotherapy in the management of bone metastases. Clin Oncol 2006;18(10): 747–60.
9. Tong D, Gillick L, Hendrickson FR. The palliation of symptomatic osseous metastases: final results of the Study by the Radiation Therapy Oncology Group. Cancer 1982;50(5):893–9.
10. Ratanatharathorn V, Powers WE, Moss WT, et al. Bone metastasis: review and critical analysis of random allocation trials of local field treatment. Int J Radiat Oncol Biol Phys 1999;44(1):1–18.
11. Ahrar K. The role and limitations of radiofrequency ablation in treatment of bone and soft tissue tumors. Curr Oncol Rep 2004;6:315–20.
12. Tam A, Ahrar K. Palliative interventions for pain in cancer patients. Semin Intervent Radiol 2007;24(4):419–29.
13. Gangi A, Basile A, Buy X, et al. Radiofrequency and laser ablation of spinal lesions. Semin Ultrasound CT MR 2005;26(2):89–97.
14. Simon CJ, Dupuy DE, Mayo-Smith MW. Microwave ablation: principles and applications. Radiographics 2005;25:569–83.
15. Gianfelice D, Gupta C, Kucharczyk W, et al. Palliative treatment of painful bone metastases with MR imaging-guided focused ultrasound. Radiology 2008; 249(1):355–63.
16. Callstrom MR, Charboneau JW, Goetz MP, et al. Painful metastases involving bone: feasibility of percutaneous CT- and US-guided radio-frequency ablation. Radiology 2002;224:87–97.

17. Callstrom MR, York JD, Gaba RC, et al. Research reporting standards for image-guided ablation of bone and soft tissue tumors. J Vasc Interv Radiol 2009;20: 1527–40.
18. Goldberg SN, Gazelle GS, Mueller PR. Thermal ablation therapy for focal malignancy: a unified approach to underlying principles, techniques, and diagnostic imaging guidance. AJR Am J Roentgenol 2000;174(2):323–31.
19. Dupuy DE, Safran H, Mayo-Smith WW, et al. Radiofrequency ablation of painful osseous metastatic disease [abstract]. Radiology 1998;209:389.
20. Carrafiello G, Lagana D, Pellegrino C, et al. Percutaneous imaging-guided ablation therapies in the treatment of symptomatic bone metastases: preliminary experience. Radiol Med 2009;114:608–25.
21. Marchal F, Brunaud L, Bazin C, et al. Radiofrequency ablation in palliative supportive care: early clinical experience. Oncol Rep 2006;15:495–9.
22. Poggi G, Gatti C, Melazzini M, et al. Percutaneous ultrasound-guided radiofrequency thermal ablation of malignant osteolyses. Anticancer Res 2003;23: 4977–84.
23. Gronemeyer DH, Schirp S, Gevargez A. Image-guided radiofrequency ablation of spinal tumors: preliminary experience with an expandable array electrode. Cancer J 2002;8(1):33–9.
24. Goetz MP, Callstrom MR, Charboneau JW, et al. Percutaneous image-guided radiofrequency ablation of painful metastases involving bone: a multicenter study. J Clin Oncol 2004;22(2):300–6.
25. Chosy SG, Nakada SY, Lee FT Jr, et al. Monitoring renal cryosurgery: predictors of tissue necrosis in swine. J Urol 1998;159:1370–4.
26. Campbell SC, Krishnamurthi V, Chow G, et al. Renal cryosurgery: experimental evaluation of treatment parameters. Urology 1998;52:29–33.
27. Hoffman NE, Bischof JC. The cryobiology of cryosurgical injury. Urology 2002; 60(2 Suppl 1):40–9.
28. Dupuy DE, Hong R, Oliver B, et al. Radiofrequency ablation of spinal tumors: temperature distribution in the spinal canal. Am J Roentgenol 2000;175: 1263–6.
29. Callstrom MR, Atwell TD, Charboneau JW, et al. Painful metastases involving bone: percutaneous image-guided cryoablation—prospective trial interim analysis. Radiology 2006;241(2):572–80.
30. Tuncali K, Morrison PR, Winalski CS, et al. MRI-guided percutaneous cryotherapy for soft-tissue and bone metastases: initial experience. Am J Roentgenol 2007; 189:232–9.
31. Bui X, Tok CH, Szwarc D, et al. Thermal protection during percutaneous thermal ablation procedures: interest of carbon dioxide dissection and temperature monitoring. Cardiovasc Intervent Radiol 2009;32:529–34.
32. Nakatsuka A, Yamakado K, Maeda M, et al. Radiofrequency ablation combined with bone cement injection for the treatment of bone malignancies. J Vasc Interv Radiol 2004;15(7):707–12.
33. Toyota N, Naito A, Kakizawa H, et al. Radiofrequency ablation therapy combined with cementoplasty for painful bone metastases. Cardiovasc Intervent Radiol 2005;28:578–83.
34. Anselmetti GC, Manca A, Chiara G, et al. Painful osteolytic metastasis involving the anterior and posterior arches of C1: percutaneous vertebroplasty with local anesthesia. J Vasc Interv Radiol 2009;20(12):1645–7.
35. Basile A, Giulano G, Scuderi V, et al. Cementoplasty in the management of painful extraspinal bone metastases: our experience. Radiol Med 2008;3(7):18–28.

36. Schaefer O, Lohrmann C, Markmiller M, et al. Technical innovation: Combined treatment of a spinal metastasis with radiofrequency heat ablation and vertebroplasty. AJR Am J Roentgenol 2003;180(4):1075–7.
37. Dupuy DE, Goldberg SN. Image-guided radiofrequency tumor ablation: challenges and opportunities – part II. J Vasc Interv Radiol 2001;12:1135–48.

Thermal Ablation of Lung Tumors

P. David Sonntag, MD[a], J. Louis Hinshaw, MD[a],*,
Meghan G. Lubner, MD[a], Christopher L. Brace, PhD[a,b],
Fred T. Lee Jr, MD[a]

KEYWORDS

• Ablation • Lung • Cancer • Thermal

Lung cancer remains the leading cause of cancer death in the United States, accounting for an estimated 29% of cancer deaths in 2009.[1] Pneumonectomy or lobectomy with hilar and mediastinal lymph node sampling is the gold standard treatment and offers the best option for cure of stage 1/2 nonsmall cell lung cancer (NSCLC).[2] Unfortunately, only 15% of patients present with stage 1/2 disease, and many of these patients do not meet the pulmonary physiologic guidelines for lobar resection.[3] In addition to lung cancer, pulmonary metastases are present in 25% to 30% of patients dying from all types of cancer.[4] For some patients with oligometastatic pulmonary disease, metastectomy is associated with an improvement in survival.[5] External beam radiation traditionally has been offered as the alternative to surgical resection for NSCLC or pulmonary metastatic disease. Unfortunately, the 5-year survival following radiation for stage 1 and 2 NSCLC remains low at 15% to 20%, with local recurrence being the most common mode of failure.[6,7] Thermal ablation offers an intriguing therapeutic option to increase local tumor control and survival in patients with early stage NSCLC or with limited metastatic disease from nonlung primaries who are not surgical candidates because of poor cardiopulmonary reserve, anatomic constraints limiting resection, failure of traditional therapies, or refusal of operative approaches.

Thermal ablation has been shown to be effective in treating tumors in bone, kidney, and liver.[8–11] Most preclinical and clinical trials have focused on demonstrating the feasibility of three modalities for pulmonary thermal ablation, namely radiofrequency (RF) ablation, microwave (MW) ablation, and cryoablation. This article discusses the unique challenges of performing thermal ablation in lung tissue and reviews the current literature regarding RF, MW, and cryoablation in the lung.

Fred T. Lee Jr, MD, is a stockholder and member of the board of directors of NeuWave Medical, Incorporated, Madison, Wisconsin. Christopher L. Brace, PhD, is a stockholder and consultant for NeuWave Medical. The other authors have nothing to disclose.

[a] Department of Radiology, University of Wisconsin, 600 Highland Avenue, Madison, WI 53792, USA
[b] Department of Biomedical Engineering, University of Wisconsin, Madison, WI, USA
* Corresponding author. Division of Abdominal Imaging, Department of Radiology, University of Wisconsin, E3/311 CSC, 600 Highland Avenue, Madison, WI 53792.
E-mail address: JHinshaw@uwhealth.org

THERMAL ABLATION IN LUNG TISSUE

Clinical success in thermal ablation depends upon the unique characteristics of the tissue being ablated. A major obstacle for all thermal ablation techniques is the heat sink effect, which describes how bloodflow or airflow through or adjacent to the target tissue can offset the applied cooling or heating, thus limiting intended tissue damage. Experimental studies with RF ablation in liver demonstrated that perfusion-mediated cooling was responsible for the smaller ablation diameters obtained in in vivo versus in vitro experiments.[12] Proximity to vessels larger than 3 mm also has been associated with increased risk of local tumor progression.[13] Thermal heat sink effects are particularly important in lung ablation, as the lungs are exposed to 100% of right heart blood flow. In addition to vascular perfusion, the lungs are uniquely composed of air-filled spaces that are constantly ventilated, resulting in a second type of heat sink analogous to an air-cooled radiator.[14]

A second factor influencing thermal ablation is the thermal conductivity of the tissue being ablated. Thermal conductivity is lower in lung than in other tissues, such as bone, liver, and kidney due to its high percentage of air by volume.[15] Lower thermal conductivity of aerated lung would be expected to limit heat transfer into tissues adjacent to solid pulmonary masses, and if true, this could prevent adequate ablation of infiltrative margins or satellite tumors at the periphery of lung lesions. Although surrounding air-filled lung may restrict heat transfer into the partially aerated peripheral portion of lesions, it may also effectively insulate the interior of lesions and create improved tumor damage via an oven- or freezer-type effect.[16,17] This has been demonstrated by animal data showing an increase in ablation zone size in implanted tumors in lung when compared with kidney.[18] A histologic study of NSCLC showed that treatment margins of 8 mm for adenocarcinoma and 6 mm for squamous cell carcinoma are necessary to cover 95% of microscopic disease.[19] The dichotomy of decreased transfer of heat to the periphery of lesions and the insulating effect of aerated lung can be an important consideration in choosing which lesions to treat and with what thermal ablation modality.

As with the liver, several investigators have attempted to overcome perfusion and ventilation heat sinks inherent to lung tissue. Ipsilateral mainstem bronchus occlusion and pulmonary artery occlusion have both been shown to significantly increase the mean volume of the ablation zone with RF ablation. Although the effect is larger with pulmonary artery occlusion, bronchial occlusion is much more practical to apply clinically.[14,20,21]

RADIOFREQUENCY ABLATION

In RF ablation, an alternating electrical current (approximately 500 KHz) with 10 to 200 W of power is applied to the target tissue via an interstitial electrode, Two to four grounding pads on the skin surface complete the electrical circuit through the body. Current conducted through tissue adjacent to the electrode leads to ion agitation, which is converted by means of friction into heat.[22] Heat generation is proportional to the current density and is attenuated exponentially with increasing distance from the electrode. As tissue is heated, predictable changes occur based on time and temperature. At temperatures between 42°C and 45°C, cells become susceptible to damage by outside agents like radiation and chemotherapy. Temperatures maintained above 46°C for a prolonged period of time (on the order of 30 to 60 minutes) cause irreversible cell damage. Between 50°C and 52°C, the time to cytotoxicity is reduced to 4 to 6 minutes. The goal of RF ablation is to achieve temperatures between 60°C and 100°C, where there is near instantaneous induction of protein coagulation with damage to cytosolic and mitochondrial enzymes and DNA–histone complexes leading to coagulative necrosis.[23,24] Conversely, temperatures above 105°C cause boiling, desiccation, vaporization, and carbonization of tissues. The resulting impedance rise limits electrical current flow, leading to reduced coagulative necrosis volumes.[25] Thus, the therapeutic temperature range for RF ablation is narrow (60°C to 100°C).

Early percutaneous RF ablation technology was able to create ablation zones only 1.6 cm in diameter.[26] Many strategies since have been developed to increase the size of RF ablations. For example, internally cooled electrodes reduce tissue charring near the electrode and permit greater energy delivery.[27] When combined with pulsed power delivery, the cooled electrodes were able to increase ablation zone size to approximately 2 cm in diameter while keeping at 17-gauge profile.[28] Clustered, deployable, and multipolar electrode designs use a different approach by increasing the effective surface area of the electrode and distributing energy delivery over a larger volume (**Fig. 1**).[29] When compared directly, it has been shown that these designs

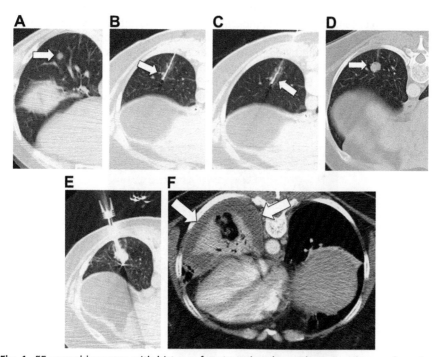

Fig. 1. 55-year-old woman with history of metastatic colorectal cancer. History of previous liver ablation, now with a new left lower lobe pulmonary metastasis. (*A*) 9 mm left lower lobe colorectal metastasis (*arrow*). (*B*) A single Cool-tip electrode was positioned, but it was somewhat eccentric in the nodule and the ground glass opacity associated with the radiofrequency ablation only partially enveloped the nodule (*arrow*), suggesting that a complete treatment was not accomplished. (*C*) 6 months later, the nodule had increased in size, and it was determined that there was local tumor progression (*arrow*). (*D*) For the retreatment, a Cool-tip cluster electrode was used to increase the power deposition, and a better technical result was achieved. (*E*) However, the increased invasiveness resulted in a large hemothorax that required chest tube placement and prolongation of her hospitalization stay. (*F*) 2-year follow-up computed tomography scan shows a small residual scar (*arrow*), but no evidence of local tumor progression.

produce potentially larger ablations than the single cooled electrode design, but often at the expense of irregular shape, protracted treatment times, or increased applicator diameter (14-gauge).[30] More recently, a system that exploits the aforementioned pulsing algorithm to switch power between multiple electrodes has been shown to increase ablation zone size while retaining a relatively spherical ablation shape.[31–33]

While most studies have focused on the performance of RF devices in liver models, some have demonstrated that multitined or multiple-electrode designs may produce more effective ablations in the lung due to their ability to spread out energy delivery.[34] However, it also has been noted that deployable designs can be more problematic to use in lung. For example, ballotable solid tumors can be difficult to penetrate with a deployable device, and some studies have described difficulty retracting the tines after treatment.[35,36]

Another strategy to overcome low tissue conductivity is by infusion of sodium chloride solutions into the targeted ablation zone.[37,38] Sodium chloride is ionic and thus improves the electrical conductivity of the surrounding tissue. Infusion during treatment also prevents charring and keeps the ablated tissue hydrated, resulting in a larger zone of ablation. However, saline infusion can produce irregular and unpredictable ablations with potentially serious complications and thus is not routinely performed.[39]

There are multiple US Food and Drug Administration (FDA)-approved RF ablation devices on the market with different performance characteristics. Examples include: the Angiodynamics 1500X RF generator with the StarBurst and Uniblate electrodes (Latham, NY, USA), the Boston Scientific RF3000 with LaVeen electrodes (Natick, MA, USA) (both of which use multitined, expandable electrodes) (**Fig. 2**) and the Covidien Cool-tip system (Boulder, CO, USA), which uses either a single straight

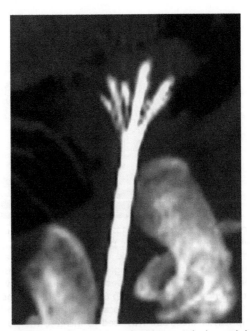

Fig. 2. A deployable array electrode positioned within a right lower lobe nonsmall cell lung cancer. Note that the increased surface area associated with this electrode allows greater power deposition, but decreased control and increased invasiveness. (*Courtesy of* Ricardo Lencioni, MD, Pisa, Italy.)

electrode, cluster of three electrodes, or up to three independent, switched straight electrodes that are actively cooled during ablation (**Fig. 3**). Importantly, these systems were all developed for use in liver, and have been applied in lung without modification. Currently, there are no devices available for clinical use optimized for treating tumors in the lung.

Animal models first were used to investigate RF ablation in normal lung tissue to develop treatment algorithms for people.[40] Human ablate-and-resect studies also were performed and, although early results were mixed, they demonstrated that RF ablation was feasible for lung tumors, ultimately leading to clinical use,[19,41] A systematic review published in 2008 summarized the literature regarding RF ablation. Among the 17 studies included in the review, the median complete necrosis rate was 90% (range: 38% to 97%) with 1-, 2- and 3-year survival rates of 63% to 85%, 55% to 65%, and 15%–46%, respectively.[42] The only prospective single-arm multicenter intent-to-treat clinical trial of RF ablation in 106 patients (33 non-small cell lung cancer, 53 colorectal cancer metastases, 20 other metastases) found promising overall and cancer-specific survival rates in these patients.[43] A summary of lung RF ablation studies is listed in **Table 1**.[34,43–51]

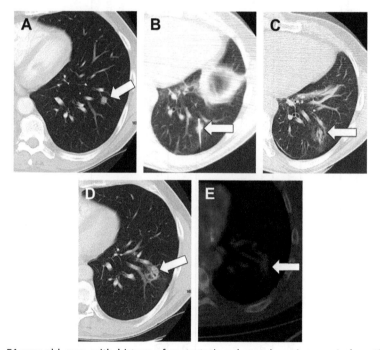

Fig. 3. 51-year-old man with history of metastatic colorectal carcinoma s/p hepatic and pulmonary resection, including right pneumonectomy, referred for radiofrequency (RF) ablation of a single left lower lobe metastatis. (*A*) 1 cm peripheral pulmonary nodule in left lower lobe (*arrow*), with no large adjacent vessels. (*B*) A single Cool-tip electrode was placed centrally in the tumor for the ablation (*arrow*). (*C*) Immediately following RF ablation, there was ground glass opacity entirely encompassing the lesion (*arrow*), consistent with a technically successful ablation. Note the small pneumothorax that resolved without treatment. (*D*) 4-month follow-up computed tomography (CT) demonstrates cavitation of the nodule (*arrow*), a favorable prognostic sign. (*E*) 14-month follow-up positron emission tomography/CT scan demonstrates parenchymal scarring, but no significant radiotracer uptake, consistent with a successful ablation.

Table 1
Summary of lung RF ablation studies

Study	Patient/Lesions	Pathology	Tumor Diameter (Mean and Range in cm)	Median Follow-Up (months)	Complications	Outcome/Comments
Akeoboshi et al, 2004[31]	31 patients/44 lesions	NSCLC, 13 Metastatic, 41	2.7 (0.7–6.0)	9.3	Ptx: 29% Ptx with chest tube: 16% Lung abscess: 6%	Complete necrosis in 69% of lesions <3 cm and 39% of lesions >3 cm
Ambrogi et al, 2006[32]	54 patients/64 lesions	NSCLC, 40 Metastatic, 24	2.4 (1.0–5.0)	23.7	Ptx: 12.7% Ptx with chest tube: 6.4%	Complete response in 61.9%, higher (69.7%) in lesions <3 cm
Belfiore et al, 2004[33]	33 patients/35 lesions	NSCLC, 35	3.5 (1.8–6.0)	—	Ptx: 9%, none with chest tube Pleural effusion: 9%	Pathologic follow-up at 6 months showed complete ablation: 36%, partial necrosis: 63% with patient pain, cough, and dyspnea scores all improved at 6 and 12 months
Gadaleta et al, 2004[34]	18 patients/40 lesions	NSCLC, 4; Metastatic, 14	3.0 (0.6–11)	9.2	Ptx: 16.7% Ptx with chest tube: 12.5%,	Complete ablation 94%
Gilliams et al, 2007[35]	37 patients/72 lesions	All metastatic	1.8 (0.4–6.6)	11.3	Major complication: 6% (ptx requiring chest tube, pleural effusion requiring drainage, tumor track seeding), Minor complication: 14% (ptx, postprocedural pain)	Recurrence in 100% of lesions >3.5 cm and 29% of lesions <3.5 cm Recurrence in 58% of lesions in direct contact with vessels and 23% in others (p>.04)
Hiraki et al, 2006[36]	128 patients/342 lesions	NSCLC 25 Metastatic, 317	1.7 (0.3–9.4)	12	—	Primary and secondary effectiveness rates: 72% and 84% at 1 y and 58% and 66% at 3 y Local progression: 27% of tumors (1–30 months), 52% of these were treated with repeat ablation Worse outcome with internally cooled electrode

Study	No. of patients/lesions	Tumor type	Size (cm)	Follow-up	Complications	Results
Lee et al, 2004[37]	30 patients/32 lesions	NSCLC, 27 Metastatic 5	5.2 (0.5–12.0)	12.5	Ptx: 23% Ptx with chest tube: 7%	Complete necrosis: 100% lesions <3 cm, 38% of lesions 3–5 cm. and 8% of lesions >5 cm Survival with complete necrosis: 19.7 months compared with 8.7 months with partial necrosis
Lencioni et al, 2004[30]	106 patients/183 lesions	NSCLC, 33 Metastatic 73	1.7 (0.5–3.4)	12	Ptx: 20.1% Ptx with chest tube 19.7%	Overall survival: 70% at 1 y and 48% at 2 y in patients with NSCLC, 89% at 1 y and 66% at 2 y in patients with colorectal metastases, and 92% at 1 y and 64% at 2 y in patients with other metastases Cancer-specific survival: 92% at 1 y and 73% at 2 y in patients with NSCLC, 91% at 1 y, and 68% at 2 y in patients with colorectal metastases Patients with other metastases: 93% at 1 y and 67% at 2 y
Yan et al, 2006[38]	55 patients	All Colorectal Metastases	2.1 (not given)	24	Ptx: 29% Ptx with chest tube: 16% Lung abscess: 4%	Median survival 33 months. 1-, 2- and 3-y actuarial survival rates were 85%, 64%, and 46% Size <3 cm was signiciantly associated with improved survival ($p<.001$)
Yasui et al, 2004[39]	35 patients/99 lesions	NSCLC, 3; Metastatic, 96	2.0 (0.3–8.0)	7.1	Ptx: 35.2% Ptx with chest tube: 4% Fever: 12%, Intraprocedureal pain 29%	Probable complete ablation: 91%

Abbreviations: NSCLC, nonsmall cell lung cancer; Ptx, pneumothorax.

There are several factors that determine the likelihood of a successful ablation, but similar to other organ systems, tumor size is one of the most important considerations.[44,49,50] Tumors less than 3.0 cm tend to be associated with complete necrosis in most cases, with less than 50% complete necrosis in tumors from 3.0 to 5.0 cm, and a low likelihood of successful ablation in tumors greater than 5.0 cm. Importantly, these studies illustrate that complete necrosis has a positive effect on survival and should be the goal of any ablative treatment.[49]

One advantage of RF ablation over surgical resection and radiation therapy is repeatability. The minimally invasive nature of percutaneous ablation allows for multiple treatment sessions on a given tumor or patient with relatively low complication risk. In fact, it has been shown that repeat treatment of local tumor progression after the primary treatment can improve survival.[34] In contrast, particularly in patients with a limited pulmonary reserve, repeat surgery is often not possible, and radiotherapy is associated with a maximum tolerated dose, which limits repeat treatment. Thus, all patients with local tumor progression should be considered for retreatment unless there is evidence of regional or distant disease.

When radiation therapy is a viable treatment option, RF ablation and external beam radiation appear to be synergistic.[52] RF ablation is most effective in the center of relatively avascular tumors, while external beam radiation and stereotactic radiosurgery are most effective at the periphery of the tumor where there is high oxygen content and a hyperthermic rim around the ablation zone. Combining the two therapies has been shown to increase survival, at no additional toxicity, as compared with radiation therapy alone, and this technique should be considered for larger tumors.[53]

In summary, RF ablation has been shown to be a suitable means of local tumor control for selected small tumors in patients with NSCLC or pulmonary metastatic disease. Pulmonary function, as measured by forced expiratory volume in the first second of respiration (FEV_1) and forced vital capacity (FVC), is well preserved following ablation, giving it a significant advantage in patients with limited pulmonary reserve.[43] Despite these promising results, RF ablation continues to be plagued by modest rates of local tumor progression, particularly in tumors greater than 3 cm and in the vicinity of larger heat sinks. Further investigation will be required to continue to improve the efficacy of this promising technique and the associated adjuvant techniques.

MW ABLATION

MW ablation is a less studied, but promising modality that may improve the efficacy of percutaneous thermal ablation in the lung. MW ablation involves the application of electromagnetic waves at frequencies of typically 915 and 2450 MHz. The alternating waves cause polar water molecules to rotate rapidly, converting the applied energy into heat and elevating tissue temperatures to cytotoxic levels.[54] As discussed previously, limitations of RF ablation include a small zone of active heating,[22] low energy delivery in high-impedance aerated or charred/desiccated tissue, and the heat sink effect.[21,55,56] In these regards MW ablation has several theoretical advantages over RF ablation. MW energy is deposited over a larger active heating zone and produces higher temperatures more quickly than is possible with RF ablation. Additionally, the electromagnetic waves associated with MW are not limited by lower thermal conductivity of lung, or the increased impedance of charred tissues.[55,57,58] MW energy also has been shown to effectively treat perivascular tissue and coagulate large vessels, with improved efficacy near heat-sinks.[59,60] Finally, multiple MW antennae can be placed and activated simultaneously, which increases ablation zone size even more than bronchial or vascular occlusion in the lung.[60,61] The performance of MW ablation is highly system dependent, and factors such as system frequency, total energy delivery, and relative phase of the alternating fields produced by each antenna can greatly affect the resulting ablation zone size. In evaluating these systems, delivered power is the most important factor for determining ablation zone size. To date, many systems have been underpowered and produce small ablation zones. The reason for this is primarily due to the inability to handle the waste heating of the antenna shaft. This heating is caused by power loss and reflected power related to impedance mismatches at the tissue/antenna interface. This is being addressed with improved cooling of the antenna shaft and better antenna design. The antenna cooling can be accomplished in several ways. The most common technique is to use water cooling similar to RF ablation systems. However, because of the higher energies and temperatures associated with MW ablation, this technique is limited. Another technique is the use of gas cooling, which is based upon the same principle as cryoablation. Because of the increased cooling power, this technique is associated with more effective cooling of the antenna shaft, allowing much higher delivered power. Further development in shaft cooling is critical to optimizing the advantages of MW ablation.

There have been several early clinical studies of MW ablation for lung tumors in people, which have shown promising rates of local control even with tumors larger than 3 cm.[62,63] The only clinically available FDA-approved MW ablation system with clinical data to date is the Evident system produced by Covidien (Boulder, CO, USA) (**Fig. 4**), but there are several other systems in development and likely to be available soon. Thus far, MW ablation has demonstrated higher pneumothorax rates than those reported in the RF ablation literature, which may be related to the large antenna size and may improve with the development of smaller antenna.[63]

Although no studies have been performed in people to compare the relative effectiveness of MW ablation and RF ablation in lung, there have been several promising studies performed in animal models. In particular, one study looked at a prototype 17 gauge internally cooled MW antennae and showed that it produced ablation zones that were 25% larger in diameter and 50% larger in cross-sectional area than the ablation zones achieved with a similarly configured internally cooled RF ablation electrode (**Fig. 5**).[57]

The current body of literature regarding clinical MW ablation in lung is limited,[63,64] but given the limitations of RF ablation regarding lung impedance, charring, and the heat sink effect, more investigation in people is warranted to determine whether the theoretical and experimental advantages of MW ablation can produce improved local control and patient survival in patients with lung tumors.

CRYOABLATION

Cryoablation causes cellular damage through a complex combination of cellular events during tissue freezing and thawing. As the temperature decreases, tissues are damaged by failed metabolism, extracellular crystallization causing cell dehydration, and finally and most severely by intracellular ice crystal formation disrupting organelles and cell membranes. Additionally, postfreezing damage occurs during thawing as ice crystals coalesce into larger crystals that disrupt cell membranes. Finally, these changes result in vascular thrombosis and stasis in the postfreezing period.[65] Given the complex nature of cellular damage that occurs with cryoablation, the protocol for lung, with its low thermal conductivity, can be expected to be somewhat different than for other tissues.[15,66] Cryoablation possesses several properties

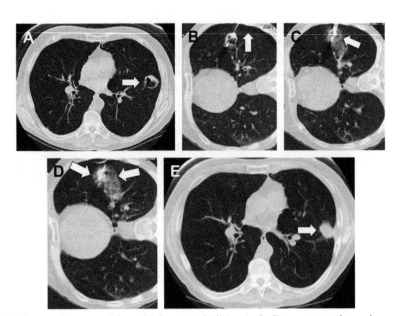

Fig. 4. 80-year-old man with multiple comorbidities, including oxygen dependence with a cavitary squamous cell carcinoma in the left lower lobe. (A) 2 cm peripheral cavitary squamous cell carcinoma in the left lower lobe (arrow). (B) Two microwave antennae were positioned within the tumor with one seen on this imaging plane. Note the small pneumothorax (arrow), which was later treated with a small-bore chest tube. (C) Due to the cavitary nature of the tumor, saline was injected into the tumor to increase the water content and thus the likelihood of heating all of the tissue. Note that after this, the tumor no longer appears cavitary (arrow). (D) Immediately after the ablation, confluent ground glass opacity develops around the tumor (arrows), indicating a combination of ablation zone and parenchymal hemorrhage. (E) 6-month follow-up computed tomography scan demonstrates a residual nodule (arrow), but without cavitation, and the patient is now 18 months post-ablation with no evidence of disease. (Courtesy of Damian Dupuy, MD, Providence, Rhode Island.)

that make it an attractive option as a thermal ablation technique. The first advantage is visualization of the ablation zone (**Fig. 6**). Radiologic–pathologic studies have shown that the ice ball visualized on computed tomography (CT) scans correlates well with the pathologic zone of ablation.[67] Second, as pulmonary fluid fills the alveolar spaces after the first freeze and thaw cycle, thermal conductivity increases 20-fold.[66] It is possible that this results in more rapid freezing and expanded ablation zones on subsequent freezing cycles.[66] Third, cryoablation preserves the collagenous architecture of the tissue being ablated, which may be particularly beneficial in treating lesions adjacent to the tracheobronchial tree and mediastinum.[68]

In the largest clinical series to date, pulmonary cryoablation was performed on 187 patients (165 primary lung, 22 metastatic), many with advanced stage disease who had failed traditional therapies. Higher technical success rates were achieved in patients with tumors less than 4 cm in diameter and peripheral tumors. Follow-up was too short to determine postprocedure survival. Of note, pulmonary cryoablation was associated with a low pneumothorax rate (12%), no procedure-related mortality, and improved quality of life scores in patients 1 week following the procedure.[69] Another study with follow-up found local tumor progression in 35% of patients, with a median time to progression of 9 months.[70] Like RF ablation, cryoablation is limited

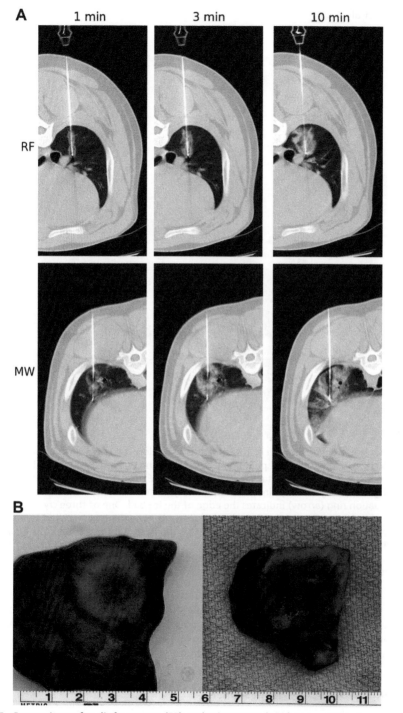

Fig. 5. Comparison of radiofrequency (RF) and microwave (MW) in a porcine lung model. (*A*) The MW ablation was associated with a more rapid and larger ablation zone than the RF ablation as shown by the development of ground glass opacity on the noncontrast computed tomography (CT) images obtained during the ablation. (*B*) The CT findings were confirmed on pathology also. (*From* Brace CL, Hinshaw JL, Laeseke PF, et al. Pulmonary thermal ablation: comparison of radiofrequency and microwave devices by using gross pathologic and CT findings in a swine model. Radiology 2009;251:705–11; with permission.)

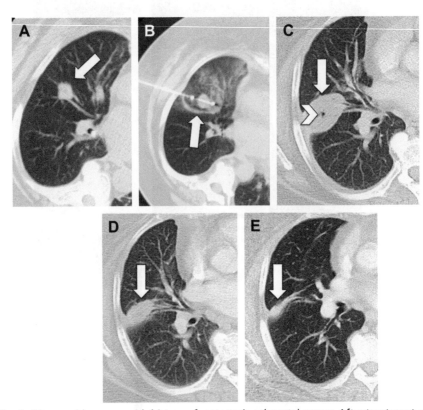

Fig. 6. 62-year-old woman with history of metastatic colorectal cancer. After treatment and resection, she had two residual pulmonary metastases and was referred for ablation. (*A*) 1.3 cm right middle lobe colorectal metastasis (*arrow*). (*B*) During pulmonary cryoablation, ground glass opacity develops in the lung parenchyma around the metastasis, and the higher attenuation ring (*arrow*) indicates the edge of the ice ball. One of three cryoprobes used for the ablation is visualized. (*C*) 1-month follow-up noncontrast computed tomography scan demonstrates expected enlargement of the apparent tumor size due to the ablation zone changes (*arrow*) and some central cavitation (*arrowhead*). (*D*) 4-month and (*E*) 12-month follow-up demonstrates progressive reduction in ablation zone size indicative of a successful ablation (*arrows*).

by the poor thermal conductivity of lung, but the ability to use numerous cryoprobes simultaneously, preservation of the collagenous tissue in airways, and a highly visible ablation zone are all advantages over heat-based therapies, particularly for larger tumors and tumors near mediastinal structures.

EVALUATION OF TREATMENT RESPONSE

Follow-up imaging after pulmonary ablation is more challenging than resection, because a both a residual mass and an ablation zone are present. In addition, ablation incites an inflammatory/cytotoxic response in adjacent normal lung tissue that appears as ground glass opacity or frank consolidation that initially increases the apparent size of the tumor. In fact, the size of the ground glass opacity surrounding the ablated lesion on immediate postablation imaging has been shown to be predictive of an effective ablation (see **Fig. 6**). One study with RF ablation suggested that a ground glass margin of at least 5 mm was required to ensure complete ablation.[71] Other investigators found that a postablation area of ground glass opacity four times the area of the ablated lesion is predictive of complete ablation.[72] The ablation zone may start to decrease in size as early as 2 to 3 weeks following ablation as tissue repair progresses, but may continue to evolve over months to years (see **Fig. 6**). Cavitation has been reported in up to 30% of patients following MW and RF ablation and is associated with effective ablation and further complicates interpretation of postablation imaging (see **Fig. 3**).

Given the apparent increase in lesion volume following ablation, the authors' follow-up protocol includes a postablation CT scan within 1 month of the procedure (to serve as a new baseline) and then contrast-enhanced CT at 3-month intervals to determine treatment response. Tumor morphology, volume, and contrast enhancement can be followed over time, and the authors consider tumors that are stable or decreasing in size and do not demonstrate more than 10 hounsfield units of contrast enhancement to be completely ablated. This method of evaluation has limitations, since some patients with incomplete treatment are not discovered until late in the follow-up period.[73]

To increase the sensitivity of detecting early recurrence some centers employ CT densitometry protocols where contrast is given, and sequential series of images are obtained at 0, 45, 180 and 300 seconds following contrast enhancement. This technique is not widely used, because it is cumbersome and not well suited to follow multiple lesions or to determine progression in complex lesions with cavitation. Positron emission tomography (PET)-CT also has been employed following ablation and can be advantageous, since it is not limited to an anatomic evaluation. Fluorodeoxyglucose (FDG) uptake should decrease in tumors as early as 2 months following ablation and nodules with a percent reduction in FDG uptake less than 60%, or an absolute SUV of 3.0 or greater at 2 months should be considered incompletely ablated and further treatment may be required.[74,75] Finally, diffusion weighted imaging (DWI) can identify differences in completely and incompletely ablated tumors, but the clinical utility of this technique is yet to be determined.[76] At this time, most clinicians follow patients with CT and use PET-CT as a problem-solving technique.

COMPLICATIONS

Although the complication rate varies and can be expected to be higher in patients who have poor underlying pulmonary reserve, a minor complication rate of approximately 50% and a major complication rate of approximately 8% can be expected. Minor complications seen after RF ablation can include: pleural effusion, pneumothorax, subcutaneous emphysema, fever, and hemoptysis, while major complications include pneumothorax requiring chest tube placement, air embolism, and pulmonary abscess.[77] Pneumothorax is the most common complication following all modalities of thermal ablation (**Fig. 7**). A median pneumothorax rate of 28% (range 4.5 to 61.1%) was reported for RF ablation in a recent meta-analysis with approximately 11% (range 3.3 to 38.9%) of these requiring chest tube placement.[42] In RF ablation, the risk of pneumothorax has been shown to be greater in patients in whom multiple lesions are treated, in patients without history of previous lung surgery, and in patients with a longer pleura-to-lesion distance.[78] In MW ablation, pneumothorax rates up to 39% have been reported.[63] This relatively high pneumothorax rate may be secondary to the larger, 14.5-gauge antenna currently available. Conversely, pneumothorax rates as low as 12% have been reported with cryoablation.[70]

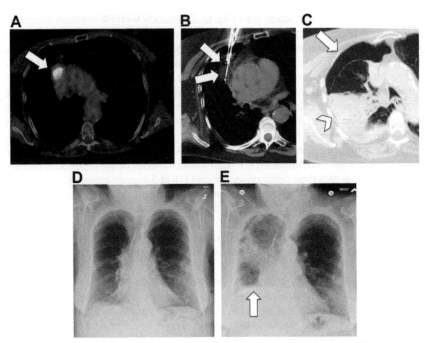

Fig. 7. 73-year-old woman with history of severe emphysema and nonsmall cell lung carcinoma in the right upper lobe. She was medically inoperable and therefore, initially treated with radiotherapy and had a good response. (*A*) 2 years after radiotherapy, she developed positron emission tomography scan-confirmed recurrent disease (*arrow*) and was not able to receive any further radiation. Therefore, she was referred for ablation. (*B*) Cryoablation was performed with 4 cryoprobes. Note low attenuation within tumor, right up to the aorta and mediastinum (*arrows*). (*C*) After the ablation, the patient developed a large and growing pneumothorax that required chest tube placement (*arrow*) and significant intraparenchymal hemorrhage (*arrowhead*), both of which contributed to significant postablation respiratory compromise. (*D*) Preablation chest radiograph showed normal relationship of the hemidiaphragms. (*E*) During the ablation, the right phrenic nerve was damaged, resulting in right hemidiaphragm paralysis, confirmed with a sniff test and seen as elevation of the right hemidiaphragm on postablation chest radiograph (*arrow*). These complications all resolved over time and in approximately 2 months, the patient returned to near her previous level of function.

Hemoptysis is a common occurrence after pulmonary ablation, but is usually low volume and self-limited. When the hemoptysis is large volume, it can be a potentially fatal event. Large-volume hemoptysis has been reported to occur in a median of 11.1% (range 3.3% to 18.2%) of patients undergoing RF ablation.[42] There has been one reported fatality following RF ablation secondary to hemoptysis; however, this patient also received brachytherapy.[79] Patients undergoing cryoablation may be at increased risk for hemoptysis, as higher rates have been reported in lung cryoablation literature, but once again, it is generally self-limited.[69,70]

Less commonly reported complications following ablation include thermal damage to the phrenic nerve, intercostal nerves and brachial plexus (see **Fig. 7**). When damaged during cryoablation, the associated symptoms tend to resolve over time. When treating lesions near the chest wall or mediastinum, an intentional pneumothorax to act as a thermal or electrical insulator can be considered to protect the intercostal or phrenic nerve.[80,81]

Microbubbles generated during thermal ablation procedures can be seen in the pulmonary veins and even the carotid artery. Although a cause of alarm when first described, this finding does not appear to be associated with adverse outcomes.[82,83] Patients undergoing thermal ablation are also at risk for air embolism and tumor track seeding similar to what is seen with needle lung biopsy.[42,84]

With MW ablation, there have been several reports of severe skin burns, possibly requiring skin grafting.[63] This is likely related to either shaft heating caused by inadequate cooling, or propagation of the MW energy along the shaft with multiple antenna ablations, resulting in nontarget tissue ablation. This issue should be addressed with the development of improved shaft cooling paradigms on future systems. An awareness of the potential complications of each of the thermal ablation modalities is an important part of preprocedural patient selection and treatment planning.

SUMMARY

The 5-year survival of all stages of NSCLC remains bleak, having only increased from 13% to 16% over the past 30 years.[1] RF ablation, MW ablation, and cryoablation are each intriguing possibilities with some track record in patients with NSCLC and pulmonary metastatic disease who are poor surgical candidates. If ablation is going to be a viable treatment for these patients, local control has to be optimized, and appropriate patient selection is key.[73] Further studies will need to address optimization of ablation protocols and should include prospective randomized trials comparing these three ablation modalities and other techniques to determine the most effective means of local tumor control in this population of patients.

REFERENCES

1. American Cancer Society. Cancer facts & figures. Atlanta (GA): The Society.
2. Deslauriers J. Current surgical treatment of nonsmall cell lung cancer 2001. Eur Respir J Suppl 2002;35:61s–70s.
3. Greene FL. American Joint Committee on Cancer. American Cancer Society. AJCC cancer staging handbook: from the AJCC cancer staging manual. 6th edition. New York: Springer; 2002.
4. Davidson RS, Nwogu CE, Brentjens MJ, et al. The surgical management of pulmonary metastasis: current concepts. Surg Oncol 2001;10:35–42.
5. Labow DM, Buell JE, Yoshida A, et al. Isolated pulmonary recurrence after resection of colorectal hepatic metastases—is resection indicated? Cancer J 2002;8:342–7.
6. Sibley GS, Jamieson TA, Marks LB, et al. Radiotherapy alone for medically inoperable stage I non-small cell lung cancer: the Duke experience. Int J Radiat Oncol Biol Phys 1998;40:149–54.
7. Sirzen F, Kjellen E, Sorenson S, et al. A systematic overview of radiation therapy effects in nonsmall cell lung cancer. Acta Oncol 2003;42:493–515.
8. Rosenthal DI, Springfield DS, Gebhardt MC, et al. Osteoid osteoma: percutaneous radiofrequency ablation. Radiology 1995;197:451–4.
9. Rossi S, Di Stasi M, Buscarini E, et al. Percutaneous radiofrequency interstitial thermal ablation in the treatment of small hepatocellular carcinoma. Cancer J Sci Am 1995;1:73–81.
10. Solbiati L, Goldberg SN, Ierace T, et al. Hepatic metastases: percutaneous radiofrequency ablation with cooled-tip electrodes. Radiology 1997;205:367–73.
11. Zagoria RJ, Traver MA, Werle DM, et al. Oncologic efficacy of CT-guided percutaneous radiofrequency ablation of renal cell carcinomas. AJR Am J Roentgenol 2007;189:429–36.

12. Goldberg SN, Hahn PF, Tanabe KK, et al. Percutaneous radiofrequency tissue ablation: does perfusion-mediated tissue cooling limit coagulation necrosis? J Vasc Interv Radiol 1998;9:101–11.
13. Gillams AR, Lees WR. Radiofrequency ablation of lung metastases: factors influencing success. Eur Radiol 2008;18:672–7.
14. Oshima F, Yamakado K, Akeboshi M, et al. Lung radiofrequency ablation with and without bronchial occlusion: experimental study in porcine lungs. J Vasc Interv Radiol 2004;15:1451–6.
15. Ponder E. The coefficient of thermal conductivity of blood and of various tissues. J Gen Physiol 1962;45:545–51.
16. Solazzo SA, Liu Z, Lobo SM, et al. Radiofrequency ablation: importance of background tissue electrical conductivity–an agar phantom and computer modeling study. Radiology 2005;236:495–502.
17. Livraghi T, Goldberg SN, Lazzaroni S, et al. Small hepatocellular carcinoma: treatment with radio-frequency ablation versus ethanol injection. Radiology 1999;210: 655–61.
18. Ahmed M, Liu Z, Afzal KS, et al. Radiofrequency ablation: effect of surrounding tissue composition on coagulation necrosis in a canine tumor model. Radiology 2004;230:761–7.
19. Ambrogi MC, Fontanini G, Cioni R, et al. Biologic effects of radiofrequency thermal ablation on nonsmall cell lung cancer: results of a pilot study. J Thorac Cardiovasc Surg 2006;131:1002–6.
20. Johansen B, Melsom MN, Flatebo T, et al. Time course and pattern of pulmonary flow distribution following unilateral airway occlusion in sheep. Clin Sci (Lond) 1998;94:453–60.
21. Anai H, Uchida BT, Pavcnik D, et al. Effects of blood flow and/or ventilation restriction on radiofrequency coagulation size in the lung: an experimental study in swine. Cardiovasc Intervent Radiol 2006;29:838–45.
22. Gazelle GS, Goldberg SN, Solbiati L, et al. Tumor ablation with radiofrequency energy. Radiology 2000;217:633–46.
23. Zervas NT, Kuwayama A. Pathological characteristics of experimental thermal lesions. Comparison of induction heating and radiofrequency electrocoagulation. J Neurosurg 1972;37:418–22.
24. Nikfarjam M, Muralidharan V, Christophi C. Mechanisms of focal heat destruction of liver tumors. J Surg Res 2005;127:208–23.
25. Goldberg SN, Gazelle GS, Halpern EF, et al. Radiofrequency tissue ablation: importance of local temperature along the electrode tip exposure in determining lesion shape and size. Acad Radiol 1996;3:212–8.
26. Goldberg SN, Gazelle GS, Dawson SL, et al. Tissue ablation with radiofrequency: effect of probe size, gauge, duration, and temperature on lesion volume. Acad Radiol 1995;2:399–404.
27. Goldberg SN. Radiofrequency tumor ablation: principles and techniques. Eur J Ultrasound 2001;13:129–47.
28. Goldberg SN, Stein MC, Gazelle GS, et al. Percutaneous radiofrequency tissue ablation: optimization of pulsed-radiofrequency technique to increase coagulation necrosis. J Vasc Interv Radiol 1999;10:907–16.
29. Goldberg SN, Solbiati L, Hahn PF, et al. Large-volume tissue ablation with radio frequency by using a clustered, internally cooled electrode technique: laboratory and clinical experience in liver metastases. Radiology 1998;209:371–9.
30. Pereira PL, Trubenbach J, Schenk M, et al. Radiofrequency ablation: in vivo comparison of four commercially available devices in pig livers. Radiology 2004;232:482–90.

31. Laeseke PF, Sampson LA, Frey TM, et al. Multiple-electrode radiofrequency ablation: comparison with a conventional cluster electrode in an in vivo porcine kidney model. J Vasc Interv Radiol 2007;18:1005–10.
32. Laeseke PF, Sampson LA, Haemmerich D, et al. Multiple-electrode radiofrequency ablation: simultaneous production of separate zones of coagulation in an in vivo porcine liver model. J Vasc Interv Radiol 2005;16:1727–35.
33. Laeseke PF, Sampson LA, Haemmerich D, et al. Multiple-electrode radiofrequency ablation creates confluent areas of necrosis: in vivo porcine liver results. Radiology 2006;241:116–24.
34. Hiraki T, Sakurai J, Tsuda T, et al. Risk factors for local progression after percutaneous radiofrequency ablation of lung tumors: evaluation based on a preliminary review of 342 tumors. Cancer 2006;107:2873–80.
35. Steinke K, King J, Glenn D, et al. Percutaneous radiofrequency ablation of lung tumors: difficulty withdrawing the hooks resulting in a split needle. Cardiovasc Intervent Radiol 2003;26:583–5.
36. Steinke K, King J, Glenn DW, et al. Percutaneous radiofrequency ablation of lung tumors with expandable needle electrodes: tips from preliminary experience. AJR Am J Roentgenol 2004;183:605–11.
37. Crocetti L, Lencioni R, Bozzi E, et al. Lung radiofrequency ablation: in vivo experimental study with low perfusion rate multitined electrodes. Cardiovasc Intervent Radiol 2008;31:610–8.
38. Lee JM, Han JK, Chang JM, et al. Radiofrequency ablation in pig lungs: in vivo comparison of internally cooled, perfusion and multitined expandable electrodes. Br J Radiol 2006;79:562–71.
39. Kim TS, Lim HK, Kim H. Excessive hyperthermic necrosis of a pulmonary lobe after hypertonic saline-enhanced monopolar radiofrequency ablation. Cardiovasc Intervent Radiol 2006;29:160–3.
40. Goldberg SN, Gazelle GS, Compton CC, et al. Radiofrequency tissue ablation of VX2 tumor nodules in the rabbit lung. Acad Radiol 1996;3:929–35.
41. Nguyen CL, Scott WJ, Young NA, et al. Radiofrequency ablation of primary lung cancer: results from an ablate and resect pilot study. Chest 2005;128:3507–11.
42. Zhu JC, Yan TD, Morris DL. A systematic review of radiofrequency ablation for lung tumors. Ann Surg Oncol 2008;15:1765–74.
43. Lencioni R, Crocetti L, Cioni R, et al. Response to radiofrequency ablation of pulmonary tumours: a prospective, intention-to-treat, multicentre clinical trial (the RAPTURE study). Lancet Oncol 2008;9:621–8.
44. Akeboshi M, Yamakado K, Nakatsuka A, et al. Percutaneous radiofrequency ablation of lung neoplasms: initial therapeutic response. J Vasc Interv Radiol 2004;15:463–70.
45. Ambrogi MC, Lucchi M, Dini P, et al. Percutaneous radiofrequency ablation of lung tumours: results in the mid-term. Eur J Cardiothorac Surg 2006;30:177–83.
46. Belfiore G, Moggio G, Tedeschi E, et al. CT-guided radiofrequency ablation: a potential complementary therapy for patients with unresectable primary lung cancer—a preliminary report of 33 patients. AJR Am J Roentgenol 2004;183:1003–11.
47. Gadaleta C, Mattioli V, Colucci G, et al. Radiofrequency ablation of 40 lung neoplasms: preliminary results. AJR Am J Roentgenol 2004;183:361–8.
48. Gillams AR, Lees WR. Analysis of the factors associated with radiofrequency ablation-induced pneumothorax. Clin Radiol 2007;62:639–44.
49. Lee JM, Jin GY, Goldberg SN, et al. Percutaneous radiofrequency ablation for inoperable nonsmall cell lung cancer and metastases: preliminary report. Radiology 2004;230:125–34.

50. Yan TD, King J, Sjarif A, et al. Percutaneous radiofrequency ablation of pulmonary metastases from colorectal carcinoma: prognostic determinants for survival. Ann Surg Oncol 2006;13:1529–37.

51. Yasui K, Kanazawa S, Sano Y, et al. Thoracic tumors treated with CT-guided radiofrequency ablation: initial experience. Radiology 2004;231:850–7.

52. Horkan C, Dalal K, Coderre JA, et al. Reduced tumor growth with combined radiofrequency ablation and radiation therapy in a rat breast tumor model. Radiology 2005;235:81–8.

53. Dupuy DE, DiPetrillo T, Gandhi S, et al. Radiofrequency ablation followed by conventional radiotherapy for medically inoperable stage I non-small cell lung cancer. Chest 2006;129:738–45.

54. Simon CJ, Dupuy DE, Mayo-Smith WW. Microwave ablation: principles and applications. Radiographics 2005;25(Suppl 1):S69–83.

55. Gabriel S, Lau RW, Gabriel C. The dielectric properties of biological tissues: II. Measurements in the frequency range 10 Hz to 20 GHz. Phys Med Biol 1996; 41:2251–69.

56. Crocetti L, Bozzi E, Faviana P, et al. Thermal ablation of lung tissue: in vivo experimental comparison of microwave and radiofrequency. Cardiovasc Intervent Radiol 2010;33(4):818–27.

57. Brace CL, Hinshaw JL, Laeseke PF, et al. Pulmonary thermal ablation: comparison of radiofrequency and microwave devices by using gross pathologic and CT findings in a swine model. Radiology 2009;251:705–11.

58. Skinner MG, Iizuka MN, Kolios MC, et al. A theoretical comparison of energy sources—microwave, ultrasound and laser—for interstitial thermal therapy. Phys Med Biol 1998;43:3535–47.

59. Yu NC, Raman SS, Kim YJ, et al. Microwave liver ablation: influence of hepatic vein size on heat-sink effect in a porcine model. J Vasc Interv Radiol 2008;19: 1087–92.

60. Brace CL, Laeseke PF, Sampson LA, et al. Microwave ablation with multiple simultaneously powered small-gauge triaxial antennas: results from an in vivo swine liver model. Radiology 2007;244:151–6.

61. Durick NA, Laeseke PF, Broderick LS, et al. Microwave ablation with triaxial antennas tuned for lung: results in an in vivo porcine model. Radiology 2008; 247:80–7.

62. Feng W, Liu W, Li C, et al. Percutaneous microwave coagulation therapy for lung cancer. Zhonghua Zhong Liu Za Zhi 2002;24:388–90.

63. Wolf FJ, Grand DJ, Machan JT, et al. Microwave ablation of lung malignancies: effectiveness, CT findings, and safety in 50 patients. Radiology 2008;247:871–9.

64. Carrafiello G, Mangini M, De Bernardi I, et al. Microwave ablation therapy for treating primary and secondary lung tumours: technical note. Radiol Med 2010;115(6):962–74.

65. Gage AA, Baust J. Mechanisms of tissue injury in cryosurgery. Cryobiology 1998; 37:171–86.

66. Hinshaw JL, Littrup PJ, Durick N, et al. Optimizing the protocol for pulmonary cryoablation: a comparison of a dual- and triple-freeze protocol. Cardiovasc Intervent Radiol 2010;33(6):1180–5.

67. Hinshaw JL. Radiology-pathology correlation of pulmonary cryoablation in a porcine model. Journal of Interventional Oncology 2009;2:113–20.

68. Littrup PJ, Mody A, Sparschu R, et al. Prostatic cryotherapy: ultrasonographic and pathologic correlation in the canine model. Urology 1994;44:175–83 [discussion: 83–4].

69. Wang H, Littrup PJ, Duan Y, et al. Thoracic masses treated with percutaneous cryotherapy: initial experience with more than 200 procedures. Radiology 2005; 235:289–98.

70. Kawamura M, Izumi Y, Tsukada N, et al. Percutaneous cryoablation of small pulmonary malignant tumors under computed tomographic guidance with local anesthesia for nonsurgical candidates. J Thorac Cardiovasc Surg 2006;131: 1007–13.

71. Anderson EM, Lees WR, Gillams AR. Early indicators of treatment success after percutaneous radiofrequency of pulmonary tumors. Cardiovasc Intervent Radiol 2009;32:478–83.

72. de Baere T, Palussiere J, Auperin A, et al. Midterm local efficacy and survival after radiofrequency ablation of lung tumors with minimum follow-up of 1 year: prospective evaluation. Radiology 2006;240:587–96.

73. Beland MD, Wasser EJ, Mayo-Smith WW, et al. Primary nonsmall cell lung cancer: review of frequency, location, and time of recurrence after radiofrequency ablation. Radiology 2010;254:301–7.

74. Okuma T, Okamura T, Matsuoka T, et al. Fluorine-18-fluorodeoxyglucose positron emission tomography for assessment of patients with unresectable recurrent or metastatic lung cancers after CT-guided radiofrequency ablation: preliminary results. Ann Nucl Med 2006;20:115–21.

75. Pua BB, Thornton RH, Solomon SB. Ablation of pulmonary malignancy: current status. J Vasc Interv Radiol 2010;21:S223–32.

76. Okuma T, Matsuoka T, Yamamoto A, et al. Assessment of early treatment response after CT-guided radiofrequency ablation of unresectable lung tumours by diffusion-weighted MRI: a pilot study. Br J Radiol 2009;82:989–94.

77. Okuma T, Matsuoka T, Yamamoto A, et al. Frequency and risk factors of various complications after computed tomography-guided radiofrequency ablation of lung tumors. Cardiovasc Intervent Radiol 2008;31:122–30.

78. Hiraki T, Tajiri N, Mimura H, et al. Pneumothorax, pleural effusion, and chest tube placement after radiofrequency ablation of lung tumors: incidence and risk factors. Radiology 2006;241:275–83.

79. Herrera LJ, Fernando HC, Perry Y, et al. Radiofrequency ablation of pulmonary malignant tumors in nonsurgical candidates. J Thorac Cardiovasc Surg 2003; 125:929–37.

80. Thornton RH, Solomon SB, Dupuy DE, et al. Phrenic nerve injury resulting from percutaneous ablation of lung malignancy. AJR Am J Roentgenol 2008;191: 565–8.

81. Lee EW, Suh RD, Zeidler MR, et al. Radiofrequency ablation of subpleural lung malignancy: reduced pain using an artificially created pneumothorax. Cardiovasc Intervent Radiol 2009;32:833–6.

82. Rose SC, Fotoohi M, Levin DL, et al. Cerebral microembolization during radiofrequency ablation of lung malignancies. J Vasc Interv Radiol 2002;13:1051–4.

83. Yamamoto A, Matsuoka T, Toyoshima M, et al. Assessment of cerebral microembolism during percutaneous radiofrequency ablation of lung tumors using diffusion-weighted imaging. AJR Am J Roentgenol 2004;183:1785–9.

84. Hiraki T, Mimura H, Gobara H, et al. Two cases of needle-tract seeding after percutaneous radiofrequency ablation for lung cancer. J Vasc Interv Radiol 2009;20:415–8.

High-Intensity Focused Ultrasound for Therapeutic Tissue Ablation in Surgical Oncology

John F. Ward, MD

KEYWORDS

- Minimally invasive ablative therapies
- High-intensity focused ultrasound • Oncologic surgery

Thermal ablative therapy has been very successful in broadening the treatment options available in many conditions that are otherwise difficult to treat using purely conventional modalities. Most thermal delivery techniques such as cryotherapy, interstitial laser, electroporation, and radiofrequency require the insertion of an applicator into the target tissue. High-intensity focused ultrasound (HIFU) is an extracorporeal, noninvasive method in which focused ultrasound beams produce complete coagulative necrosis at the target lesions through intact skin without surgical exposure or instrumentation. Lynn and colleagues[1] described the possibility of using ultrasound to carry out destructive surgery of this nature as early as 1942. Because HIFU does not require an internal applicator, there is no risk for puncture-related bleeding or needle track dissemination of malignant cells, and it is effective even when the tumor is poorly perfused (as opposed to electroconductive treatments that require a relatively uniformly hydrated treatment volume). Sound waves enter the body over a broad surface area with diffuse energy insufficient to cause thermal injury, then pass to a single focal point where their combined energy, enhanced by constructive sonic wave interference, is capable of elevating tissue temperature to lethal levels (65°–85°C). It is only in the past 20 years that technology has enabled this concept be safely developed; however, a substantial amount of work remains to refine current technology platforms to allow for treatment throughout the entire body.

THE PHYSICS OF HIGH-INTENSITY FOCUSED ULTRASOUND

Sound is vibration. In physics, the term "ultrasound" applies to all acoustic energy (longitudinal, mechanical wave) with a frequency above the audible range of human

Department of Urology, University of Texas MD Anderson Cancer Center, PO Box 301439, Houston, TX 77230-1439, USA
E-mail address: jfward@mdanderson.org

Surg Oncol Clin N Am 20 (2011) 389–407
doi:10.1016/j.soc.2010.11.009
1055-3207/11/$ – see front matter © 2011 Elsevier Inc. All rights reserved.

surgonc.theclinics.com

hearing: between about 20 and 20,000 Hz. Sounds with frequencies higher than this range are termed ultrasound. Planar ultrasound waves deposit clinically insignificant energy as they travel through tissues.

All medical applications of ultrasound make use of the piezoelectric effect (**Fig. 1**A, B). The piezoelectric effect is a reversible process in which certain solid materials (notably crystals and some ceramics) will have internal generation of a mechanical force when an electrical charge is applied (converse piezoelectric effect). These materials will also exhibit the direct piezoelectric effect, namely the generation of an electrical charge when a mechanical force is applied. When a series of electrical pulses (ie, an alternating electrical current) is passed through a piezoelectric crystal, mechanical waves are created that propagate away from the crystal. As the waves pass across an interface of different tissues, the speed of the wave propagation will change. Each time the speed of sound changes, ie, different tissue density, some of it will be reflected, or echoed, back to the crystal, and some will continue propagating forward. When an echo returns, it vibrates the crystal, creating an electric current that can be analyzed and processed to construct an image. Typical diagnostic ultrasound has a single crystal that rapidly alternates between transmission and listening modes. Diagnostic sonographic scanners typically operate in the frequency range of 2 to 18 MHz, the choice of frequency being a trade-off between spatial resolution of the image and imaging depth: lower frequencies produce less resolution but image deeper into the body.

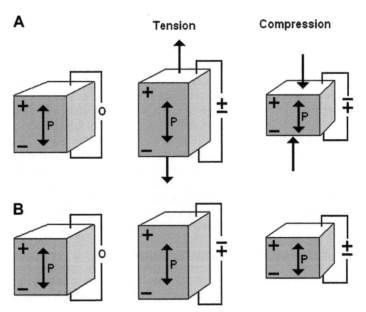

Fig. 1. (*A*) Direct piezoelectric effect: Certain single crystal materials when mechanically strained, or when the crystal is deformed by the application of an external stress, will generate an electric charge on the surface of the crystal. When the direction of the strain reverses, the polarity of the electric charge is reversed. (*B*) Converse piezoelectric effect: When a piezoelectric crystal is placed in an electric field, the crystal exhibits strain, ie, the dimensions of the crystal change. When the direction of the applied electric field is reversed, the direction of the resulting strain is reversed.

Mechanical index (MI) is the peak rarefaction pressure of an ultrasound longitudinal wave and is a standard measure of the acoustic output in a diagnostic ultrasound system. It is also an important concept to understand how an ultrasonic wave can produce desirable tissue damage. As MI increases, microbubbles are generated within the tissue as the ultrasonic wave physically deforms the tissue. If MI is elevated enough, rupture of these microbubbles will occur. Diagnostic ultrasound becomes therapeutic ultrasound when the peak MI, intended to occur at the focal zone of the ultrasound beam, nears or exceeds this threshold. For diagnostic imaging, intermediate acoustic power (0.1 <MI <0.5) is used, which deposits very little, nondisruptive energy into tissue. High-intensity focused ultrasound, as opposed to planar ultrasound, exceeds these diagnostic acoustic powers and deposits a much larger amount of energy (5000 and 100,000 times greater than those of diagnostic ultrasound) into the tissue.[2] The increased wave intensity is focused, either geometrically or electronically (phased array), onto a single point. When the acoustic power at this focus point is sufficiently high, cavitation (microbubbles forming and interacting with the ultrasound field) will occur. Microbubbles produced in the field oscillate and grow (owing to factors including rectified diffusion), and eventually implode (inertial or transient cavitation). During the inertial cavitation, very high temperatures will occur inside the bubbles (65° to 85°C), destroying the tissue by coagulation necrosis. The internal cavitation is followed by a sudden and violent collapse of the microbubble that results in a shock wave, which causes additional mechanical damage to the tissue.[3–6] Stable cavitation is the oscillation of existing microbubbles in the tissue and is not associated with a violent collapse and dispersion of energy. Microbubble oscillations can result in sheering forces and viscous-damping heating. Although stable cavitation is currently avoided during the procedure, there is some experimental evidence that stable cavitation may be able to enhance tissue ablation during HIFU and is being further investigated.[7,8]

During HIFU, a reproducible but small volume of ablation is created for each pulse of energy. The geometry of each ablation volume is an ellipsoid, and the size of the ellipsoid is a function of crystal geometry. Through sequential movements of the applicator, the targeted volume is systematically ablated. Stacking these pulses of high intensity ultrasound will achieve this tissue destruction in as large or small of a volume as planned and desired (**Fig. 2**).[9] Tissues beyond the elementary ablation volume may heat slightly with more conduction perpendicular to the long axis of the elementary lesion than parallel to it. No ischemic infarction is produced by this technique. Cooling

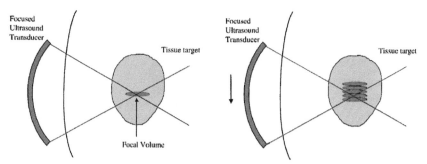

Fig. 2. Stacked treatment volumes allow precise painting of the targeted area with ablative ultrasonic waves. The volume of tissue ablated (length, height, and width) are dependent upon the delivery device but can be adjusted some by the operator for individualized therapy.

intervals are placed between each sonication so that the tissue anterior and, to a lesser extent, posterior to the focal spot cool between sonications, allowing further sonications to be placed closer to the first one without any damage to the intervening tissues.[10] The passage of the HIFU beam through the tissues depends on the same physical factors as conventional diagnostic ultrasound. In other words, gas will reflect the HIFU beam and may cause areas of high heat build up at tissue-gas interfaces that must be avoided. Bone and calcifications will absorb HIFU energy very avidly, potentially shielding structures immediately behind them from heating but may also cause heat build up at the bone–soft tissue interface.

HIFU TARGETING AND MONITORING

Two methods are available to visualize, target, and monitor the tissue designated for destruction with HIFU: diagnostic ultrasound and magnetic resonance imaging (MRI). However, no single universally adhered method of using focused ultrasound (FUS) has yet emerged.

Diagnostic Ultrasound

The most common method to target and monitor HIFU therapy uses conventional diagnostic ultrasound transducers.[11] Two separate crystals (therapeutic and diagnostic) can be packaged into one instrument (**Fig. 3**). This allows for real-time monitoring of the target and a visual estimation of the acoustic coupling and any potential confounders of successful therapeutic HIFU delivery (air, bone, calcifications). This method allows a reasonable amount of flexibility in the targeting, but it does have several substantial drawbacks.

First, to fit both crystals into a single applicator, the applicator is larger and heavier than traditional diagnostic ultrasound probes. Size is a particular problem when designing applicators to be placed within natural orifices (eg, the esophagus, rectum, urethra, or uterus) rather than for transcutaneous application (eg, the liver, kidney, or pancreas). A smaller crystal has a smaller potential depth of the focal zone. As such, this can limit the ability to treat a greater depth of tissue penetration and limits treatment to organs proximal to the applicator (eg, smaller prostates). Diagnostic ultrasound also has low spatial resolution, limiting its accuracy for targeting (in comparison with MR imaging). In addition, when there is bowel and air in the vicinity, it may be hard to visualize the details of adjacent structures around these gas-containing portions, as well as behind them, so that targeting may be limited.[12] Finally,

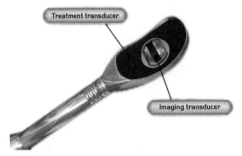

Fig. 3. Single transrectal probe containing 2 ultrasonic crystals: one for the delivery of HIFU, the second for targeting and monitoring the treatment in real time.

thermal mapping is difficult with ultrasound. Under ultrasound observation, the tissue temperatures are estimated through observation of changes in the tissue echogenicity and induction of microbubbles and cavitation. Although there are a variety of techniques becoming gradually available that may improve the thermal resolution of ultrasound, these techniques remain quite cumbersome. Despite these relative drawbacks, HIFU with ultrasound guidance has been used to treat many patients, particularly in the Far East, in a variety of applications and shows substantial promise in these areas.[13–15]

Magnetic Resonance Imaging

Developing HIFU machinery that works in the extremely hostile environment of an MR scanner is a substantial technical achievement.[16–18] No ferromagnetic material may be used and radiofrequency leakage from electrical components will cause substantial MR image degradation. Simple motion of the transducer has to be accomplished by MR-compatible means, such as the use of piezoelectric motors rather than conventional electric motors. Substantial filtering of radiofrequency leakage together with shielding of electric connections must be used to limit interference with imaging.

Imaging with MR offers excellent visualization of the full extent of tumor within its tissue structure and depicts the boundary of soft tissues very clearly. It is precisely this ability that is so useful in the targeting of HIFU and where diagnostic ultrasound guidance alone is most problematic. Additionally, MR allows real-time thermal resolution with high spatial resolution (**Fig. 4**). Therefore, thermal maps are rapidly and easily acquired with MR and are accurate to $\pm 2°C$ using conventional phase shift imaging.[19] Several MRI parameters are temperature sensitive and allow detection of small temperature elevations before any induced irreversible tissue damage.[20] Thus, the focus can be located at relatively low powers, and the accuracy of targeting can be verified. In addition, by using temperature-sensitive MRI sequences, focal temperature elevations and effective thermal doses may be estimated.[21–23] An added advantage is that MRI is often used for preoperative and postoperative assessment of the targeted area so that consistent imaging platforms can be used to monitor therapeutic results. However, MRI is expensive and bulky. The treatment time is also prolonged, because despite its imaging advantages, the acquisition of images is much more time consuming than ultrasound.

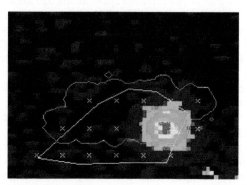

Fig. 4. Thermal map from real-time MRI imaging during uterine fibroid ablation with HIFU.

THE HIFU EQUIPMENT
Magnetic Resonance–Guided Focused Ultrasound

Gadolinium-enhanced T1-weighted images clearly show the extent of necrosis following an HIFU treatment.[24] MRI has also been used to guide HIFU treatment and to monitor temperature changes during HIFU (see **Fig. 4**).[25]

Currently, only one commercially available MR-compatible HIFU machine is available (ExAblate 2000, Insigtec, Haifa, Israel), although several other prototypes are currently being tested (Phillips Healthcare, Amsterdam, The Netherlands).

The ExAblate 2000 system consists of 4 components, which all work in synergy. These are the MR scanner, the HIFU table containing the transducer and water bath, the electronic components driving the system, and the HIFU workstation. The latter links to the MR workstation and allows user interaction. To date, this system works only on the General Electric (Fairfield, CT, USA) MRI scanner platform. The HIFU table is identical to the conventional MR table, with the addition of a built-in transducer and water bath, and electronic connections. The current machinery contains a 211-phased array element within a water bath. The transducer may be moved by its robotic system to any position in the water bath, and the depth of focus can be varied electronically to allow great flexibility of positioning. The transducer frequency is variable, ranging from 0.9 to 1.4 MHz.

Recently, the combination of planar ultrasound transducers under rotational control with active MR temperature feedback that can produce conformal spatial patterns of thermal damage within the prostate gland has been described.[26,27] To achieve this, a device containing the piezoelectric treatment crystal is inserted into the urethra and delivers high-intensity ultrasound energy to adjacent prostate tissue.[28] MR imaging is used during treatment to measure the spatial temperature distribution in the prostate and surrounding tissues noninvasively.[27–30] This unique capability to measure the temperature distribution in the prostate gland continuously during treatment enables adaptive therapy delivery that can compensate for changes in blood flow or ultrasound properties of the prostate gland that are known to occur during heating.[31,32] In addition, quantitative knowledge of the amount of heating in surrounding tissues can be used to protect critical structures (rhabdosphincter, erectile nerves, rectum) from thermal damage. A prototype system for MRI-guided transurethral ultrasound therapy within a conventional closed-bore MR environment is now being developed by Profound Medical Inc (Toronto, Canada).[26,33,34]

Ultrasound-Guided HIFU for Prostate Cancer Treatment

Current transducers for transrectal prostate applications use single-focus transducers that are moved mechanically. There are 2 HIFU technologies currently used for the treatment of prostate cancer, although neither one is yet approved by the Food and Drug Administration (FDA). The first developed was the Ablatherm (Edap-Technomed, Lyon, France). Subsequently, Focus Surgery Inc (Indianapolis, IN, USA) developed a system called the Sonablate. The Ablatherm consists of a specific bed containing the ablation technology upon which the patient lies in a lateral position. For the Sonablate system, the procedure is conducted in a lithotomy position.

The Ablatherm includes 3 predefined treatment protocols with specifically designed energy parameters depending on the clinical use (Primary therapy, HIFU retreatment, and failure after prior radiation) (**Fig. 5**A, B). The Sonablate uses a single treatment protocol in which the operator manually adapts the power. This "visually directed" HIFU treatment is based on gray-scale ultrasonographic changes observed during treatment that allow the operator to change the power level for each HIFU pulse.[35]

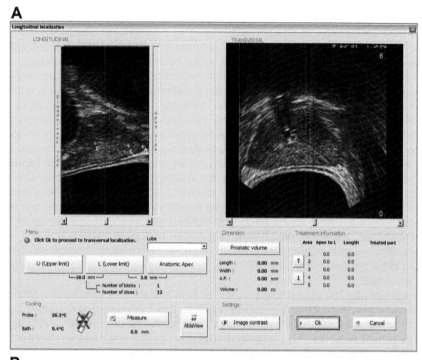

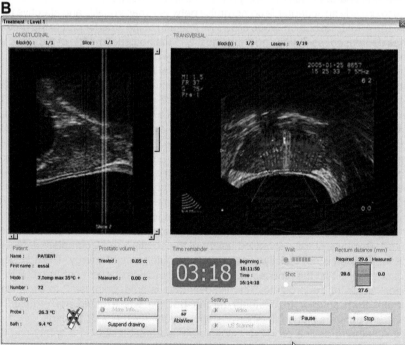

Fig. 5. (*A*) Prostate treatment planning on the Ablatherm allows for transverse and sagittal transrectal ultrasonography and treatment targeting. (*B*) Prostate treatment on the Ablatherm. Each "shot" ablates a very defined, targeted area of tissue. These "shots" are sequentially stacked to ablate the desired volume of tissue.

The underlying science and technology of both systems is identical but differences from different schools of thought with regard to how to best design the optimal HIFU treatment system have led to very different machines. Specifically, the differences arise in how the manufacturers choose optimal ultrasonic frequencies and powers, as well as differences on the optimal method for proceeding through the treatment plan. These differences have in turn led to differences in image quality and treatment-induced cavitation. Increasing the frequency increases the incidence of cavitation, increases image resolution near the ultrasound crystal, but reduces ultrasound penetration. The fundamental physical constraint in the design of a transducer is the fact that it must be inserted into the rectum during treatment. The physical size and shape of the ultrasound transducer determines where the energy can be focused.

The Ablatherm uses separate crystals for imaging (7.5 MHz) and treatment (3.0 MHz). Thus, the dependence of image resolution is removed from the equation when ablation is occurring. Imaging probes for standard prostate applications tend to range from 5.0 MHz to 7.5 MHz, with higher frequency probes creating higher quality images. The real-time 7.5-MHz probe used by the Ablatherm creates a very high-quality image throughout the prostate and a 3.0-MHz treatment probe was determined to be the best for treatment.[36] Thus, optimal values are used for both imaging and treatment.

The Sonablate 500 uses a single crystal for both imaging and treatment: a concave rectangular element cut from a spherical crystal surface that has a central 10-mm diameter segment used for imaging. There is no need to change probes between imaging and treatment; however, this constrains the probe to be of a single frequency, as probe frequency is characteristic of the crystal. An operating frequency of 4 MHz was determined to provide an acceptable compromise between image quality and effective treatment. The 4-MHz resolution probe allows for imaging of the anterior part of the prostate but has decreased resolution and image quality in the posterior margin of the gland and the rectal wall in comparison with higher frequency ultrasound probes.

The Ablatherm uses a single treatment probe that has a focal point 45 mm from the crystal. The 3-MHz probe creates an ablation volume size that is adjustable from 24.0 (anterior to posterior) $\times$ 1.7 $\times$ 1.7 mm (total volume = 36 mm³) down to 19.0 $\times$ 1.7 $\times$ 1.7 mm (total volume = 29 mm³). The intent is that a single pulse will result in an ablation that extends the entire anterior to posterior height of the prostate. This strategy has the advantage that only one focus is needed to treat the entire height of the gland, but given that prostates are not uniform in height (the base is taller than the apex), it can result in the ablation of some tissue beyond the anterior margin of the prostate.

The Sonablate probe is composed of 2 different crystals with different focal lengths. This is accomplished by having 2 crystals placed back to back within the probe, one with a 3-cm focal length and the other with a 4-cm focal length. The discrete ablation volume of both these crystals is 10 (anterior to posterior) $\times$ 2 $\times$ 2 mm (total volume = 21 mm³). Because of the decreased height of the ablation zone, complete anterior to posterior ablation is not usually possible with a single pulse of energy. The advantage to this strategy is that the reduced ablation volume provides better conformation to the anterior margin of the prostate. The disadvantage is time, because 2 to 3 planes of treatment from anterior to posterior throughout the whole gland are required, as most every prostate has an anterior posterior height in excess of 10 mm.

The Ablatherm device provides many safety features, including a safety ring that stabilizes the rectum wall, a permanent control of the distance between the therapy transducer and the rectal wall, and a patient motion detector. The Sonablate requires a permanent presence of the physician during the procedure to control the adequacy between what was planned and what is done.

Ultrasound-Guided Transcutaneous HIFU

Currently, only Haifu Technology Company (Chongqing, China) produces an ultrasound guided/monitored HIFU system for the treatment of a variety of benign and malignant solid organ tumors (uterine fibroid, benign breast neoplasm, benign tumors of soft tissues, malignant bone tumor, liver cancer, sarcoma of soft tissue, renal cancer, breast cancer, bladder caner, pancreatic cancer, tumor metastasis).[37-39] This system consists of 3 selectable therapeutic transducers and a real-time imaging transducer. The transducers are mounted in a water reservoir with the beam axis directed upward, and the patients positioned above the transducers in a prone or decubitus position. Although certified by the European Union for the treatment of benign and malignant soft tissue tumors, this technology is not yet available in North America even through clinical trials, and is currently available in 3 European and 4 Asian centers. Theoretically, this system would be less costly and time consuming than MR-guided devices.

THERAPEUTIC APPLICATIONS OF HIFU
Uterine Fibroids

Adenomyosis (leiomyomas, uterine fibroids) is a common gynecologic disorder of women during their reproductive lives. It is characterized by the presence of ectopic endometrial glands and stroma in the myometrium.[40,41] Initial studies using this technology to treat uterine fibroids were limited to fibroids of a maximum 10-cm diameter, as this was part of an early FDA-sanctioned study.[42-44] Patients were enrolled who had fibroids that could be easily accessed via a suitable acoustic window through the anterior abdominal wall without a substantial amount of bowel interposed between the uterus and the abdominal wall. In some instances, bladder filling may create an acoustic window but this is not always the case. Similarly, it has become evident that scars in the pathway of the HIFU beam are problematic, as the dense collagenous, fibrous, avascular nature of the scar absorbs ultrasound avidly, and causes local heating and possibly even burning of the skin. Initial studies have shown an excellent improvement in symptoms as measured by dedicated uterine fibroid symptom severity scores in nearly 80% of patients.[45]

However, many fibroids are much larger than 10 cm in diameter and these are often associated with much greater symptoms. These patients are treated with gonadotropin-releasing hormone (GnRH) agonists for 3 months, which usually results in a significant degree of fibroid shrinkage (40% volume reduction), enabling conventional HIFU ablation.[46] In addition, it seems that the effects of each HIFU sonication are potentiated by the GnRH agonist pretreatment.[47] A study examining 50 patients with fibroids all greater than 10 cm (10–20 cm) indicated that patients treated in this manner had a symptomatic response equal to that of the previous study when only fibroids smaller than 10 cm were treated.[46] This type of adjuvant therapy applied to this HIFU technique has greatly increased the range of fibroids that can be treated in this way. Initial groups of treated patients were only those who had completed their family; however, some of these patients have become pregnant and delivered healthy babies without any complications to the pregnancy.[48]

Breast Cancer

The intention of using HIFU in the treatment of breast cancer is to try to replace conventional surgery with a completely noninvasive procedure maintaining efficacy and reducing the cosmetic impact of lumpectomy. This would allow patients to have an outpatient treatment with no associated surgical scars and to replace open surgical procedures such as lumpectomy and wide local excision. The overall treatment for breast cancer would otherwise be as normal in terms of radiotherapy, drug treatments, and sentinel node biopsy. Studies are at an early stage, but, in a study of 30 patients in Japan treated with HIFU followed by a lumpectomy of the treated area, 97% of malignant cells in the treated area were destroyed by this procedure.[49,50] This high percentage is extremely promising and may exceed the percentage of cells considered to be removed by conventional lumpectomy.[51] Studies continue in this area but these early results appear promising and currently expanded versions of the study are ongoing. Development of similar protocols where patients receive HIFU without subsequent surgery and the patient is followed over a period of time using detailed imaging criteria to measure the response are also now under way.

Liver and Pancreas

There is a wealth of experience in the literature describing the use of percutaneous thermal destructive devices, such as laser, radiofrequency, or microwave probes, in the treatment of local liver disease owing to primary or secondary hepatic tumors.[52] Success rates in these areas are highly promising with very low morbidity and reduced inpatient stay in comparison with conventional hepatic surgery.[53] In this field, HIFU has the potential of eliminating the invasiveness of current ablative treatment of hepatic masses and the complications of placing needles and probes into an often-times more widely diseased liver.

Hepatic MR-guided focused ultrasound (MRgFUS) does have some technical issues that still need to be overcome: most of the liver is covered by the ribcage and the footprint of the HIFU beam from the current transducer is relatively wide. The ribs absorb the HIFU, preventing a reliable focused target from being achieved in the liver and there can be substantial rib heating produced. This can cause not only damage to the underlying bone, but also potential heating and burning of the overlying skin. Currently, only areas of the liver that are below the rib line or in the mid line and not covered by the ribs, can be treated. Voluntary respiratory motion of the liver may prevent consistent repeated sonications to the target zone owing to unpredictable movement of the liver. An MR-compatible ventilator coupled to the HIFU applicator has allowed the HIFU machine to sonicate at the same position of the patient's diaphragm so that a targeted area can be more precisely treated.[54]

Bone

Radiotherapy is the most common conventionally used treatment in patients with painful primary or metastatic bone tumors. Unfortunately, a proportion of patients continue to have pain despite the additional use of other conventional therapies, such as hormonal manipulation and chemotherapy. Several groups have attempted to use percutaneous thermal ablation techniques similar to those in the liver and other areas of the body to treat these conditions. Callstrom and colleagues[55] describe 62 patients treated with this form of percutaneous thermal therapy using radiofrequency ablation techniques with very effective improvement in pain scores following just a single treatment. Bone also displays piezoelectric properties and will absorb HIFU avidly, rapidly inducing periosteum heating. Interestingly, palliation of pain has been much more effective when the periphery of the target lesion is treated rather than its center, which when treated alone has resulted in poorer pain relief. It is postulated, therefore, that the periosteum is the primary site of pain induction in these conditions. Therefore, HIFU may be easily applied to wide areas of the periosteum using a broader portion of the beam rather than just the small focal spot.[56] This type of modified application allows treatment to encompass relatively large areas of the periosteum with each sonication. Therefore, HIFU in bone may provide a noninvasive 1-stop outpatient treatment of painful bone lesions with highly effective pain control, without the need for longer courses and multiple attendances, as is usually required for radiotherapy. Similarly, radiotherapy failures may also be treated with this type of approach in an effective manner.

Brain

Although presence of bone in the ultrasound beam path contraindicates most applications of FUS, early work at 2 sites in the world is finding that FUS can be deposited within the brain through the closed skull. This requires complex computational calculation of calvarial thickness and curvature along the potential lines of sonication, but it is becoming clear that destructive energy can be focused through the closed skull into target areas within the brain to destroy tissues.[57,58] The potential of achieving trackless surgical destruction of abnormal brain lesions through a closed skull under MR guidance holds tremendous therapeutic potential; however, many problems in this very complex application still need to be solved.

Prostate Cancer

HIFU has experienced its widest application in the treatment of patients with prostate cancer; both the patient undergoing primary treatment as well as those in need of local salvage therapy after failed radiotherapy (**Table 1**).[59–63]

Originally introduced 15 years ago for the treatment of benign prostatic hypertrophy, its potential for the minimally invasive treatment of localized prostate cancer was recognized in short course to be more significant.[64] The National Institute for Clinical Excellence (NICE) in the United Kingdom evaluated HIFU in 2005 and found that there was sufficient evidence to recommend its use for the treatment of localized prostate cancer. Subsequently, in 2008, NICE recommended the use of HIFU in controlled clinical trials or when patients are entered into a registry and closely followed to determine its long-term efficacy.[65] This change in statement was put forth by the council not as a negative guidance, but rather a positive one in which they felt the reported outcomes so far were good; continued good study and reporting of long-term outcomes will be necessary to receive the full endorsement of this council.[65] The French Association of Urology (FAU) and the Association of Italian Urologists (AURO) both recommend HIFU as standard treatment for patients with localized disease who are unsuitable for or who failed radiation, or who are unsuitable for surgery.[66] The European Association of Urology guidelines, however, state HIFU is "investigational or experimental."[67] In the United States, the American Urological Association (AUA) has not provided guidance on HIFU for prostate cancer treatment because it is currently not approved by the FDA for treatment of prostate cancer outside ongoing investigational trials. As more studies provide longer-term disease-free rates and treatment-associated morbidity, it is expected that more positive consensus recommendations on the use of HIFU for localized prostate cancer will emerge.

In 1995, Madersbacher and colleagues[68] used the Sonablate 200 in 10 patients with localized prostate cancer. In 1996, Gelet and colleagues[69] reported a preliminary experience with an Ablatherm prototype in almost the same indications. From these first articles to the contemporary series, several publications with both devices have confirmed the HIFU efficacy as a primary procedure with short- and midterm results and, importantly, increasing information on the effects of prostate HIFU on quality of life.[59,61,70,71] End points available in these series are either freedom from biochemical (serum prostate-specific antigen [PSA]) recurrence, with highly variable definitions making comparisons between series and devices difficult at best, biopsy data, or

Table 1
Outcomes following high-intensity focused ultrasound

Study	Device	Patients, n	Clinical Stage	Mean Pre-HIFU PSA, ng/mL	Mean or Median Follow-up, mo	Negative Biopsies, %	Mean or Median PSA Nadir, ng/mL	DFSR, Criteria
Uchida et al[86]	S	63	T1c-2b N0 M0	11.2	22.3	87	0.5	74% at 3 y (ASTRO 1997)
Chaussy and Thuroff[87]	A	271	T1-2 Nx/0 M0	8.3	14.8	84.6	0	82.1% (ASTRO 1997)
Lee et al[88]	A	58	T1-2 Nx/0 M0	10.9	14	N/A	0.2	69% at 14 mo (ASTRO 97 + Biopsy)
Poissonnier et al[89]	A	227	T1-2 Nx/0 M0	6.99	27	86	0.1	N/A
Vallancien et al[90]	A	30	T1-2 Nx/0 M0	7	20	83	0.9	N/A
Thuroff et al[91]	A	402	T1-2 Nx/0 M0	10.9	13.1	87.2	0.6	N/A
Blana et al[70]	A	140	T1-2 Nx/0 M0	7	76.8	86.4	0.16	69% at 7 y (ASTRO 2005)
Crouzet et al[61]	A	803	T1-2 Nx/0 M1	9.1	42	77.9	0.25	83% Low risk, 72% Intermediate risk, 68% High risk (ASTRO 2005 + Biopsy)

Abbreviations: A, Ablatherm integrated imaging (EDAP-TMS SA, Vaulx en Velin, France); ASTRO, The American Society for Therapeutic Radiology and Oncology; DFSR, disease-free survival rate; HIFU, high-intensity focused ultrasound; PSA, prostate-specific antigen; S, Sonablate 500 (Focus Surgery, Indianapolis, IN, USA).

a combination of both. On the basis of combined pathologic or biochemical outcomes, the estimated 5-year disease-free survival rate following primary HIFU is between 66% and 78% (see **Table 1**).

Crouzet and colleagues[61] recently reported the largest multicenter, retrospective analysis of cancer-specific outcomes following primary HIFU. Outcomes from 803 patients with at least 2 years of follow-up treated between 1993 and 2007 at 6 European centers are included in this analysis. Most patients harbored low- to intermediate-risk prostate cancer according to risk group assignment (40.2%, 46.3%, and 13.5% of patients, respectively). Mean follow-up was 42 ± 33 months. All patients were regularly assessed with baseline and post-HIFU PSA levels at 3, 6, and 12 months, and then every 6 months. Post-HIFU biopsies regardless of PSA value at 6 months were available in 589 patients (73.3%). Biopsies were negative in 459 patients (77.9%) and positive in 130 patients (22.1%). In case of positive prostate biopsy during follow-up without evidence of metastasis, HIFU retreatment was reperformed. The negative biopsy rate was statistically significantly different ($P = .003$) for men with low-, intermediate-, and high-risk disease: 84.9%, 73.5%, and 72.0%, respectively. Mean PSA nadir was 1.0 ± 2.8 ng/mL with 54.3% reaching a nadir of 0.3 ng/mL or less. The overall and cancer-specific survival rates at 8 years were 89% and 99%, respectively. The metastasis-free survival rate at 8 years was 97%. Additional treatment-free survival rates were 84%, 68%, and 54% ($P<.001$) for low-, intermediate-, and high- risk patients, respectively. PSA nadir was a major predictive factor for HIFU success defined as negative biopsies, stable PSA, and no additional therapy.

FUTURE HIFU APPLICATIONS
HIFU Combined with Chemotherapeutics

Experimental studies have demonstrated the potential of synergistic inhibitory effect of the HIFU plus cytotoxic chemotherapy.[72] ThermoDox (Celsion Corporation, Columbia, MD, USA) is a proprietary heat-activated liposomal encapsulation of doxorubicin that is currently in Phase I-III clinical investigation for treatment of hepatic and breast carcinomas. Hyperthermia of the HIFU releases the entrapped doxorubicin from the liposome. This delivery technology enables high concentrations of doxorubicin to be deposited preferentially in a targeted tumor with minimal systemic side effects.

For primary liver cancer, a 600-patient global Phase III study at 75 clinical sites under an FDA Special Protocol Assessment is under way with ThermoDox. The study is designed to evaluate the efficacy of ThermoDox in combination with thermal ablation compared with patients who receiving thermal ablation alone. The primary end point for the study is progression-free survival and the trial is 75% enrolled at this writing. For recurrent chest wall breast cancer, ThermoDox is being evaluated in a pivotal Phase I/II open-label, dose-escalating trial that is designed to measure durable local complete response at the tumor site. Approximately 100 patients across the United States are expected to be enrolled by the first half of 2011.

Treatment-Induced Immunology

Impaired immune function is a factor in the development and progression of human tumors. In most cancer patients, lymphocyte-mediated immunity fails to control the development and growth of the primary tumor, and cannot prevent local recurrence and metastasis after conventional therapies. Spontaneous regression of tumor metastases has been reported after ablation of primary lesions, particularly following cryosurgical procedures. This suggests that during the process of the necrotic tissue resorption by the host, active immunity to the tumor tissue can develop, but this has been an unpredictable response in humans.[73–75]

After HIFU, a large amount of tumor debris remains in situ. This debris contains tumor antigens and heat shock proteins (HSP), such as HSP60,[76] HSP27,[77] HSP72 and HSP73,[78] and HSP70.[79] Local infiltration of activated dendritic cells in the debris of HIFU-treated breast cancer has been demonstrated.[80]

The Chongqing China group has been most active in the investigation of immune responses induced through HIFU ablation of tumors. They have recently demonstrated that the remaining tumor debris activates dendritic cells and that dendritic cells loaded with HIFU-ablated tumor debris elicit greater lymphocyte proliferation and induce tumor-specific cytotoxicity through activation of cytotoxic T-cell lymphocytes (CTLs).[81,82] Immune protection of the peripheral blood lymphocytes purified from HIFU-treated H22 tumor-bearing mice was also observed. Long-term follow-up results, such as survival rate, tumor extinction rate, and metastatic rate, were significantly better in the HIFU group than in the sham-HIFU and control groups. These findings support the potential that HIFU-activated CTLs could have therapeutic potential as adoptive immunotherapy for homogeneous tumors.

A growing body of clinical reports has suggested that this systemic immune response observed in the mouse model is also present in cancer patients following HIFU ablation. Rosberger and colleagues[83] reported 5 consecutive cases of posterior choroidal melanoma treated with HIFU. Patient immune function was monitored by determination of T-cell helper/suppressor (CD4/CD8) ratios immediately before and approximately 1 week after HIFU treatment. Three patients had abnormal and 2 patients had normal CD4/CD8 ratios before treatment. One week after treatment, the ratio in 2 patients reverted to normal, whereas another was noted to have a 37% increase in his CD4 cells relative to his CD8 cells. Two patients with initially normal CD4/CD8 demonstrated no significant change postoperatively. Wang and Sun used multiple-session HIFU (average: 8.1 sessions; range: 2–12 sessions) to treat 15 patients with late-stage pancreatic cancer.[84] Changes in natural killer (NK) cell activity and T lymphocytes and subsets were observed in 10 patients before and after HIFU treatment. The results showed that the average values of NK cell, CD3+, CD4+, and CD4+/CD8+ ratios in peripheral blood increased after HIFU in 10 patients. A statistically significant difference was observed in only NK cell activity before and after HIFU treatment ($P<.05$).

Wu and colleagues[85] observed changes in circulating NK cells, T lymphocytes, and subsets in patients with solid malignancy treated with a single session of ablative HIFU. There was a mix of solid tumors (6 osteosarcoma [Enneking Stage IIB 4, IIIB 2]; 5 hepatocellular carcinoma [TNM Stage III 3, IV 2], and 5 renal cell carcinoma [TNM Stage III 2, IV 3]). T lymphocyte and subsets, B lymphocytes, and NK cells in the peripheral blood were measured in these patients on the day before HIFU and 7 to 10 days after HIFU. The results showed a significant increase in the population of CD4+ lymphocytes ($P<.01$) and the ratio of CD4+/CD8+ ($P<.05$) in the blood circulation of cancer patients after HIFU treatment. The abnormal levels of CD3+ lymphocytes returned to normal in 2 patients, CD4+/CD8+ ratio in 3 patients, CD19+ lymphocytes in 1 patient, and cytotoxic NK in 1 patient respectively, in comparison with the values in the control group.

SUMMARY

High-intensity focused ultrasound as a trackless, noninvasive method of ablating tissue has been a concept with potential for more than 60 years. It is only in the past 10 to 15 years that technological advances in both the delivery system and the monitoring systems have allowed us to begin to truly explore this potential clinically. Although unique technical challenges remain to be overcome, this ablative technique has been successfully applied in nearly all regions of the body, even some hidden by dense bone. The possibility that HIFU may be synergistic in ways that other ablative therapies are not, with both chemotherapeutics and immune system modifiers, positions HIFU for further investigations into multidisciplinary, individualized therapy unique to the patient.

REFERENCES

1. Lynn J, Zwemer R, Chick A, et al. New method for the generation and use of focused ultrasound in experimental biology. J Gen Physiol 1942;26:179.
2. Haar GT, Coussios C. High intensity focused ultrasound: physical principles and devices. Int J Hyperthermia 2007;23:89.
3. Barnett SB, ter Haar GR, Ziskin MC, et al. Current status of research on biophysical effects of ultrasound. Ultrasound Med Biol 1994;20:205.
4. Hill CR, ter Haar GR. Review article: high intensity focused ultrasound—potential for cancer treatment. Br J Radiol 1995;68:1296.
5. Linke CA, Carstensen EL, Frizzell LA, et al. Localized tissue destruction by high-intensity focused ultrasound. Arch Surg 1973;107:887.
6. Magin RL, Fridd CW, Bonfiglio TA, et al. Thermal destruction of the canine prostate by high intensity microwaves. J Surg Res 1980;29:265.
7. Curiel L, Chavrier F, Gignoux B, et al. Experimental evaluation of lesion prediction modelling in the presence of cavitation bubbles: intended for high-intensity focused ultrasound prostate treatment. Med Biol Eng Comput 2004;42:44.
8. Kennedy JE, Ter Haar GR, Cranston D. High intensity focused ultrasound: surgery of the future? Br J Radiol 2003;76:590.
9. Foster RS, Bihrle R, Sanghvi NT, et al. High-intensity focused ultrasound in the treatment of prostatic disease. Eur Urol 1993;23(Suppl 1):29.
10. ter Haar G. Therapeutic ultrasound. Eur J Ultrasound 1999;9:3.
11. ter Haar G. Ultrasound focal beam surgery. Ultrasound Med Biol 1995;21:1089.
12. Hynynen K, Freund W, Cline H, et al. A clinical, noninvasive, MR imaging-monitored ultrasound surgery method. Radiographics 1996;16:185.
13. Illing RO, Kennedy JE, Wu F, et al. The safety and feasibility of extracorporeal high-intensity focused ultrasound (HIFU) for the treatment of liver and kidney tumours in a Western population. Br J Cancer 2005;93:890.
14. Wu F. Extracorporeal high intensity focused ultrasound in the treatment of patients with solid malignancy. Minim Invasive Ther Allied Technol 2006;15:26.
15. Wu F, Wang ZB, Zhu H, et al. Feasibility of US-guided high-intensity focused ultrasound treatment in patients with advanced pancreatic cancer: initial experience. Radiology 2005;236:1034.
16. Cline HE, Schenck JF, Hynynen K, et al. MR-guided focused ultrasound surgery. J Comput Assist Tomogr 1992;16:956.
17. Jolesz FA, Hynynen K. Magnetic resonance image-guided focused ultrasound surgery. Cancer J 2002;8(Suppl 1):S100.
18. McDannold N, Tempany CM, Fennessy FM, et al. Uterine leiomyomas: MR imaging-based thermometry and thermal dosimetry during focused ultrasound thermal ablation. Radiology 2006;240:263.
19. McDannold NJ, Jolesz FA. Magnetic resonance image-guided thermal ablations. Top Magn Reson Imaging 2000;11:191.

20. Hynynen K, Pomeroy O, Smith DN, et al. MR imaging-guided focused ultrasound surgery of fibroadenomas in the breast: a feasibility study. Radiology 2001;219: 176.
21. Hynynen K, Damianou C, Darkazanli A, et al. The feasibility of using MRI to monitor and guide noninvasive ultrasound surgery. Ultrasound Med Biol 1993;19:91.
22. Vimeux FC, De Zwart JA, Palussiere J, et al. Real-time control of focused ultrasound heating based on rapid MR thermometry. Invest Radiol 1999;34:190.
23. Visioli AG, Rivens IH, ter Haar GR, et al. Preliminary results of a phase I dose escalation clinical trial using focused ultrasound in the treatment of localised tumours. Eur J Ultrasound 1999;9:11.
24. Rouviere O, Lyonnet D, Raudrant A, et al. MRI appearance of prostate following transrectal HIFU ablation of localized cancer. Eur Urol 2001;40:265.
25. de Senneville BD, Mougenot C, Moonen CT. Real-time adaptive methods for treatment of mobile organs by MRI-controlled high-intensity focused ultrasound. Magn Reson Med 2007;57:319.
26. Chopra R, Burtnyk M, Haider MA, et al. Method for MRI-guided conformal thermal therapy of prostate with planar transurethral ultrasound heating applicators. Phys Med Biol 2005;50:4957.
27. Hazle JD, Diederich CJ, Kangasniemi M, et al. MRI-guided thermal therapy of transplanted tumors in the canine prostate using a directional transurethral ultrasound applicator. J Magn Reson Imaging 2002;15:409.
28. Diederich CJ, Stafford RJ, Nau WH, et al. Transurethral ultrasound applicators with directional heating patterns for prostate thermal therapy: in vivo evaluation using magnetic resonance thermometry. Med Phys 2004;31:405.
29. Chen JC, Moriarty JA, Derbyshire JA, et al. Prostate cancer: MR imaging and thermometry during microwave thermal ablation—initial experience. Radiology 2000;214:290.
30. Peters RD, Chan E, Trachtenberg J, et al. Magnetic resonance thermometry for predicting thermal damage: an application of interstitial laser coagulation in an in vivo canine prostate model. Magn Reson Med 2000;44:873.
31. Wagrell L, Sundin A, Norlen B. Intraprostatic blood-flow changes during Prosta-Lund feedback treatment measured by positron emission tomography. J Endourol 2005;19:873.
32. Xu LX, Zhu L, Holmes KR. Blood perfusion measurements in the canine prostate during transurethral hyperthermia. Ann N Y Acad Sci 1998;858:21.
33. Chopra R, Baker N, Choy V, et al. MRI-compatible transurethral ultrasound system for the treatment of localized prostate cancer using rotational control. Med Phys 2008;35:1346.
34. Tang K, Choy V, Chopra R, et al. Conformal thermal therapy using planar ultrasound transducers and adaptive closed-loop MR temperature control: demonstration in gel phantoms and ex vivo tissues. Phys Med Biol 2007;52:2905.
35. Illing RO, Leslie TA, Kennedy JE, et al. Visually directed high-intensity focused ultrasound for organ-confined prostate cancer: a proposed standard for the conduct of therapy. BJU Int 2006;98:1187.
36. Sanghvi NT, Hawes RH. High-intensity focused ultrasound. Gastrointest Endosc Clin N Am 1994;4:383.
37. Dong X, Yang Z. High-intensity focused ultrasound ablation of uterine localized adenomyosis. Curr Opin Obstet Gynecol 2010;22:326.
38. Jung SE, Cho SH, Jang JH, et al. High-intensity focused ultrasound ablation in hepatic and pancreatic cancer: complications. Abdom Imaging 2010. [Epub ahead of print].

39. Orsi F, Zhang L, Arnone P, et al. High-intensity focused ultrasound ablation: effective and safe therapy for solid tumors in difficult locations. AJR Am J Roentgenol 2010;195:W245.

40. Byun JY, Kim SE, Choi BG, et al. Diffuse and focal adenomyosis: MR imaging findings. Radiographics 1999;19:S161.

41. Ota H, Igarashi S, Hatazawa J, et al. Is adenomyosis an immune disease? Hum Reprod Update 1998;4:360.

42. Hindley J, Gedroyc WM, Regan L, et al. MRI guidance of focused ultrasound therapy of uterine fibroids: early results. AJR Am J Roentgenol 2004;183:1713.

43. Lenard ZM, McDannold NJ, Fennessy FM, et al. Uterine leiomyomas: MR imaging-guided focused ultrasound surgery—imaging predictors of success. Radiology 2008;249:187.

44. Tempany CM, Stewart EA, McDannold N, et al. MR imaging-guided focused ultrasound surgery of uterine leiomyomas: a feasibility study. Radiology 2003;226:897.

45. Stewart EA, Rabinovici J, Tempany CM, et al. Clinical outcomes of focused ultrasound surgery for the treatment of uterine fibroids. Fertil Steril 2006;85:22.

46. Smart OC, Hindley JT, Regan L, et al. Gonadotrophin-releasing hormone and magnetic-resonance-guided ultrasound surgery for uterine leiomyomata. Obstet Gynecol 2006;108:49.

47. Smart OC, Hindley JT, Regan L, et al. Magnetic resonance guided focused ultrasound surgery of uterine fibroids—the tissue effects of GnRH agonist pre-treatment. Eur J Radiol 2006;59:163.

48. Rabinovici J, Inbar Y, Eylon SC, et al. Pregnancy and live birth after focused ultrasound surgery for symptomatic focal adenomyosis: a case report. Hum Reprod 2006;21:1255.

49. Furusawa H, Namba K, Nakahara H, et al. The evolving non-surgical ablation of breast cancer: MR guided focused ultrasound (MRgFUS). Breast Cancer 2007;14:55.

50. Gianfelice D, Khiat A, Amara M, et al. MR imaging-guided focused US ablation of breast cancer: histopathologic assessment of effectiveness—initial experience. Radiology 2003;227:849.

51. Mendez JE, Lamorte WW, de Las Morenas A, et al. Influence of breast cancer margin assessment method on the rates of positive margins and residual carcinoma. Am J Surg 2006;192:538.

52. Livraghi T, Meloni F, Morabito A, et al. Multimodal image-guided tailored therapy of early and intermediate hepatocellular carcinoma: long-term survival in the experience of a single radiologic referral center. Liver Transpl 2004;10:S98.

53. Mack MG, Straub R, Eichler K, et al. Breast cancer metastases in liver: laser-induced interstitial thermotherapy—local tumor control rate and survival data. Radiology 2004;233:400.

54. Kopelman D, Inbar Y, Hanannel A, et al. Magnetic resonance-guided focused ultrasound surgery (MRgFUS): ablation of liver tissue in a porcine model. Eur J Radiol 2006;59:157.

55. Callstrom MR, Charboneau JW, Goetz MP, et al. Image-guided ablation of painful metastatic bone tumors: a new and effective approach to a difficult problem. Skeletal Radiol 2006;35:1.

56. Liberman B, Gianfelice D, Inbar Y, et al. Pain palliation in patients with bone metastases using MR-guided focused ultrasound surgery: a multicenter study. Ann Surg Oncol 2009;16:140.

57. Hynynen K, McDannold N, Clement G, et al. Pre-clinical testing of a phased array ultrasound system for MRI-guided noninvasive surgery of the brain—a primate study. Eur J Radiol 2006;59:149.

58. McDannold N, Clement GT, Black P, et al. Transcranial magnetic resonance imaging-guided focused ultrasound surgery of brain tumors: initial findings in 3 patients. Neurosurgery 2010;66:323.

59. Berge V, Baco E, Karlsen SJ. A prospective study of salvage high-intensity focused ultrasound for locally radiorecurrent prostate cancer: early results. Scand J Urol Nephrol 2010;44:223.

60. Blana A, Walter B, Rogenhofer S, et al. High-intensity focused ultrasound for the treatment of localized prostate cancer: 5-year experience. Urology 2004; 63:297.

61. Crouzet S, Rebillard X, Chevallier D, et al. Multicentric oncologic outcomes of high-intensity focused ultrasound for localized prostate cancer in 803 patients. Eur Urol 2010;58:559–66.

62. Poissonnier L, Murata FJ, Chapelon JY, et al. [Indications, techniques and outcomes of high-intensity focused ultrasound (HIFU) for the treatment of localized prostate cancer]. Ann Urol (Paris) 2007;41:237 [in French].

63. Uchida T, Shoji S, Nakano M, et al. Transrectal high-intensity focused ultrasound for the treatment of localized prostate cancer: eight-year experience. Int J Urol 2009;16:881.

64. Gelet A, Chapelon JY, Bouvier R, et al. Local control of prostate cancer by transrectal high intensity focused ultrasound therapy: preliminary results. J Urol 1999; 161:156.

65. Guidelines on prostate cancer: diagnosis, staging and therapy. In: Association of Italian Urologists. 10th Auroline. Ligure (Italy); 2008.

66. Rebillard X, Soulie M, Chartier-Kastler E, et al. High-intensity focused ultrasound in prostate cancer: a systematic literature review of the French Association of Urology. BJU Int 2008;101:1205.

67. Heidenreich A, Aus G, Bolla M, et al. EAU guidelines on prostate cancer. Eur Urol 2008;53:68.

68. Madersbacher S, Pedevilla M, Vingers L, et al. Effect of high-intensity focused ultrasound on human prostate cancer in vivo. Cancer Res 1995;55:3346.

69. Gelet A, Chapelon JY, Bouvier R, et al. Treatment of prostate cancer with transrectal focused ultrasound: early clinical experience. Eur Urol 1996;29:174.

70. Blana A, Murat FJ, Walter B, et al. First analysis of the long-term results with transrectal HIFU in patients with localised prostate cancer. Eur Urol 2008;53:1194.

71. Shoji S, Nakano M, Nagata Y, et al. Quality of life following high-intensity focused ultrasound for the treatment of localized prostate cancer: a prospective study. Int J Urol 2010;17:715.

72. Paparel P, Curiel L, Chesnais S, et al. Synergistic inhibitory effect of high-intensity focused ultrasound combined with chemotherapy on Dunning adenocarcinoma. BJU Int 2005;95:881.

73. Bayjoo P, Rees RC, Goepel JR, et al. Natural killer cell activity following cryosurgery of normal and tumour bearing liver in an animal model. J Clin Lab Immunol 1991;35:129.

74. Miya K, Saji S, Morita T, et al. Experimental study on mechanism of absorption of cryonecrotized tumor antigens. Cryobiology 1987;24:135.

75. Muller LC, Micksche M, Yamagata S, et al. Therapeutic effect of cryosurgery of murine osteosarcoma—influence on disease outcome and immune function. Cryobiology 1985;22:77.

76. Hu Z, Yang XY, Liu Y, et al. Release of endogenous danger signals from HIFU-treated tumor cells and their stimulatory effects on APCs. Biochem Biophys Res Commun 2005;335:124.

77. Madersbacher S, Grobl M, Kramer G, et al. Regulation of heat shock protein 27 expression of prostatic cells in response to heat treatment. Prostate 1998;37:174.

78. Kramer G, Steiner GE, Grobl M, et al. Response to sublethal heat treatment of prostatic tumor cells and of prostatic tumor infiltrating T-cells. Prostate 2004;58: 109.

79. Wu F, Wang ZB, Cao YD, et al. Expression of tumor antigens and heat-shock protein 70 in breast cancer cells after high-intensity focused ultrasound ablation. Ann Surg Oncol 2007;14:1237.

80. Xu ZL, Zhu XQ, Lu P, et al. Activation of tumor-infiltrating antigen presenting cells by high intensity focused ultrasound ablation of human breast cancer. Ultrasound Med Biol 2009;35:50.

81. Deng J, Zhang Y, Feng J, et al. Dendritic cells loaded with ultrasound-ablated tumour induce in vivo specific antitumour immune responses. Ultrasound Med Biol 2010;36:441.

82. Zhang Y, Deng J, Feng J, et al. Enhancement of antitumor vaccine in ablated hepatocellular carcinoma by high-intensity focused ultrasound. World J Gastroenterol 2010;16:3584.

83. Rosberger DF, Coleman DJ, Silverman R, et al. Immunomodulation in choroidal melanoma: reversal of inverted CD4/CD8 ratios following treatment with ultrasonic hyperthermia. Biotechnol Ther 1994;5:59.

84. Wang X, Sun J. High-intensity focused ultrasound in patients with late-stage pancreatic carcinoma. Chin Med J (Engl) 2002;115:1332.

85. Wu F, Wang ZB, Lu P, et al. Activated anti-tumor immunity in cancer patients after high intensity focused ultrasound ablation. Ultrasound Med Biol 2004;30:1217.

86. Uchida T, Ohkusa H, Yamashita H, et al. Five years experience of transrectal high-intensity focused ultrasound using the Sonablate device in the treatment of localized prostate cancer. Int J Urol 2006;13:228.

87. Chaussy C, Thuroff S. The status of high-intensity focused ultrasound in the treatment of localized prostate cancer and the impact of a combined resection. Curr Urol Rep 2003;4:248.

88. Lee HM, Hong JH, Choi HY. High-intensity focused ultrasound therapy for clinically localized prostate cancer. Prostate Cancer Prostatic Dis 2006;9:439.

89. Poissonnier L, Chapelon JY, Rouviere O, et al. Control of prostate cancer by transrectal HIFU in 227 patients. Eur Urol 2007;51:381.

90. Vallancien G, Prapotnich D, Cathelineau X, et al. Transrectal focused ultrasound combined with transurethral resection of the prostate for the treatment of localized prostate cancer: feasibility study. J Urol 2004;171:2265.

91. Thuroff S, Chaussy C, Vallancien G, et al. High-intensity focused ultrasound and localized prostate cancer: efficacy results from the European multicentric study. J Endourol 2003;17:673.

Index

Note: Page numbers of article titles are in **boldface** type.

Surg Oncol Clin N Am 20 (2011) 409–416
doi:10.1016/S1055-3207(10)00142-0
1055-3207/11/$ – see front matter © 2011 Elsevier Inc. All rights reserved.

surgonc.theclinics.com